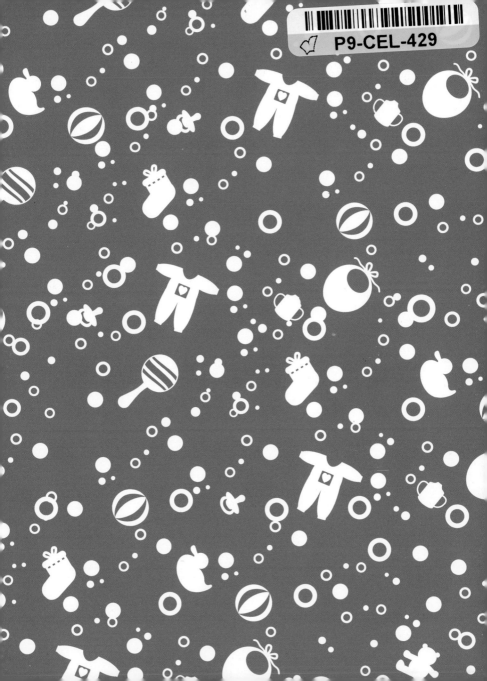

P9-CEL-429

Preggatinis™

Mixology for the Mom-to-Be

Natalie Bovis-Nelsen
aka The Liquid Muse

Photographs by Claire Barrett

gpp
life

Guilford, Connecticut
An imprint of The Globe Pequot Press

To buy books in quantity for corporate use
or incentives, call **(800) 962-0973**
or e-mail **premiums@GlobePequot.com.**

Copyright © 2009 by Natalie Bovis-Nelsen

ALL RIGHTS RESERVED. No part of this book may be reproduced or transmitted in any form by any means, electronic or mechanical, including photocopying and recording, or by any information storage and retrieval system, except as may be expressly permitted in writing from the publisher. Requests for permission should be addressed to The Globe Pequot Press, Attn: Rights and Permissions Department, P.O. Box 480, Guilford, CT 06437.

GPP Life is an imprint of The Globe Pequot Press

Preggatinis™ is a trademark of Natalie Bovis-Nelsen.

"Mediterranean Layer Dip with Toasted Pita Triangles" on p. 105, from *The Most Decadent Diet Ever!* by Devin Alexander, copyright © 2008 by Devin Alexander. Published by Broadway Books, a division of Random House, Inc. Reprinted with permission.

Design by Diana Nuhn
Spot art throughout © Shutterstock

Library of Congress Cataloging-in-Publication Data
Bovis-Nelsen, Natalie.
  Preggatinis : mixology for the mom-to-be / Natalie Bovis-Nelsen, aka The Liquid Muse ; photographs by Claire Barrett.
      p. cm.
  ISBN 978-1-59921-454-2
  1. Non-alcoholic cocktails. 2. Pregnant women. I. Title.
  TX815.B745 2009
  641.8'75—dc22

                                                2008031759

Printed in China

10 9 8 7 6 5 4 3

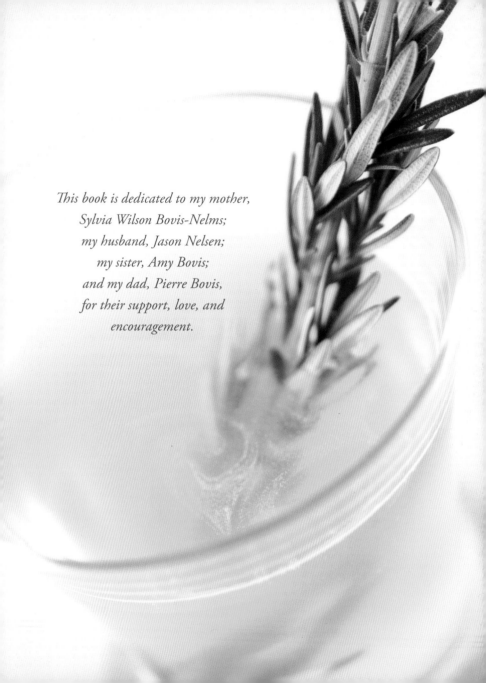

*This book is dedicated to my mother,
Sylvia Wilson Bovis-Nelms;
my husband, Jason Nelsen;
my sister, Amy Bovis;
and my dad, Pierre Bovis,
for their support, love, and
encouragement.*

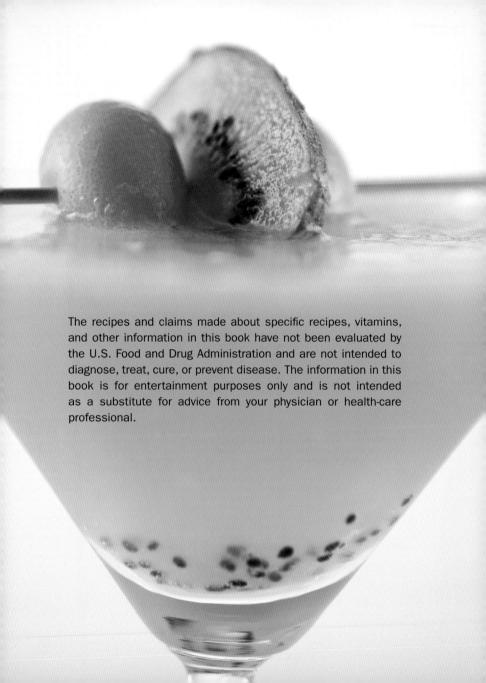

The recipes and claims made about specific recipes, vitamins, and other information in this book have not been evaluated by the U.S. Food and Drug Administration and are not intended to diagnose, treat, cure, or prevent disease. The information in this book is for entertainment purposes only and is not intended as a substitute for advice from your physician or health-care professional.

ACKNOWLEDGMENTS

I would like to acknowledge the following people, for whom I have heartfelt gratitude:

My girlfriends, who share an enthusiasm for cocktails (even nonalcoholic ones).

My community of fellow cocktail bloggers, mixologists, bartenders, and Sipsters (people who read The Liquid Muse Blog).

Claire Barrett, whose gorgeous photos bring my recipes to life.

Lilly Ghahremani, who gave me deadlines when I needed them and then went to bat to make this project a reality.

And Mary Norris, who understood my vision, heard my voice, and gently guided me through the thrilling and daunting process of writing my first book!

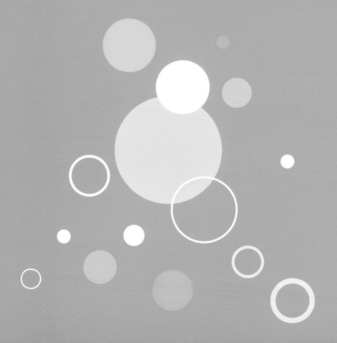

Contents

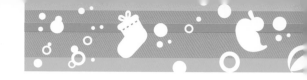

Prelude to a Preggatini

Welcome to one of the biggest decisions of your life . . . to give up cocktails for nine months! Nonalcoholic Preggatinis are designed to make that transition easy—and even enjoyable. Created with the fun and stylish modern mom-to-be in mind, Preggatinis retain the glitz of any alcoholic "tini" drink. They are colorful and exotic and presented in fancy stemware. Best of all, you'll have a blast shaking, stirring, and muddling when you "belly up" to your own Preggatini home bar.

As The Liquid Muse (www.theliquid muse.com), I create cocktail recipes for all sorts of upscale events and liquor launches. Therefore, I approach the Preggatini the way I would a traditional cocktail. Not to be confused with the goopy, syrupy, unappetizing "mocktails" you may have encountered in the past, a Preggatini is created from freshly squeezed juices, fresh fruit or vegetables, herbs, and homemade syrups. Although I don't write the word *organic* in each recipe, you can assume that it is implied for all ingredients.

The tools of the trade, mixers, and basic rules for making a balanced drink don't change, with or without alcohol. Many of these recipes turned out so well, that readers may have a hard time kicking the Preggatini habit post-baby! So, I've included "de-virginize" options for dads, nonpregnant friends, and you, once you've had the baby and your doctor gives the green light. Hold on to this book and make notes along the way, because long after the little one's arrival, the recipes and sidebar tips within will serve you well!

I occasionally list premade flavored ingredients for the sake of your convenience. And in some recipes, I specify certain brands. These are purely my preferences or suggestions. Please feel free to make your own syrups and purees, and substitute your own favorite brands of non-alcoholic wine or beer.

Thanks to the glamorization of pregnancy by today's celebrities, the baby bump has become a declaration of sexy femininity and, yes, a fashion statement. A stylish pregnancy is part of the modern mom movement and *Preggatinis* is *the* how-to book for sipping your way through this special time when you are the star, the VIP—when the world seems to revolve around your belly! Enjoy being the new "It" girl because, with your journey toward motherhood the Preggatini Party has just begun. . . .

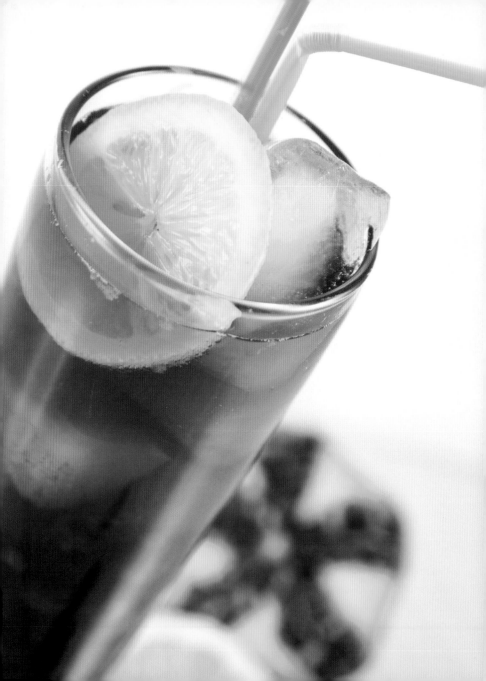

Part 1

The nursery is baby's nest, haven, safety zone. In the coming months you'll pick the perfect crib, changing table, and hanging mobile. You'll stock up on diapers, wet wipes, and onesies. You'll buy bottles, bags, and baby baubles. Baby's "happy place" will be ready and waiting. Meanwhile, mommy's happy place is the Preggatini Home Bar!

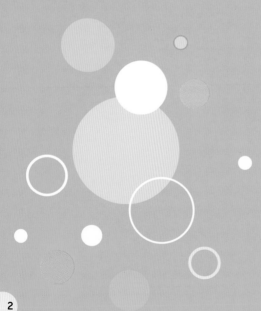

The Tools of the Trade

Can an artist paint without a brush? Can a guitarist strum a melody without an instrument? Now apply that philosophy to making a cocktail. (Yes, even a nonalcoholic one!) Here are some basic tools every home bar needs.

BAR SPOON: This looks like a teaspoon with a very long stem, ideal for stirring ingredients in a tall glass.

CITRUS PRESS: A one-step tool for squeezing the juice from a lemon or lime.

COCKTAIL SHAKER: There are many kinds of shakers out there, and the prettier ones aren't always the most functional. A plain old Boston shaker is the most professional alternative. It comes in two parts, the mixing glass and the tin lid. I like this one because you can see the ingredients in the mixing glass as you

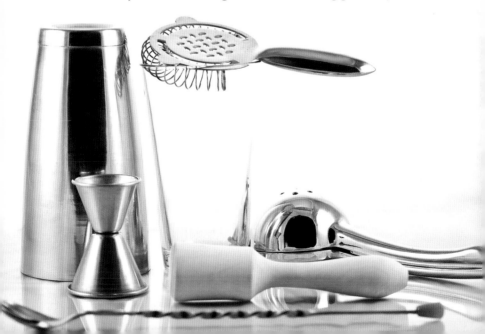

make the drink. When you secure the tin lid on top of the glass, the shaker will seal. When you're ready to open it up, give it a good whack on the side where the two glasses meet to unseal it.

JIGGER: This is used for measuring liquid ingredients. The larger side typically measures a "jigger," or 1½ ounces, and the smaller side measures a "pony," or 1 ounce.

MUDDLER: This is basically a pestle with a longer handle so it can reach to the bottom of a mixing glass. Don't pound and smash the fruit or fresh herbs in the bottom of the mixing glass, but rather "muddle" them by gently squeezing the muddler down upon them in a rotating motion. This will release the oils and juices, integrating the natural flavors.

PARING KNIFE AND CUTTING BOARD: You will be chopping, slicing and peeling fruits, vegetables, and herbs, so a sharp knife and cutting board will be integral.

STRAINER: If you buy a Boston shaker, it will not have a built-in strainer, so choose one that fits well over the opening of the mixing glass. It is best to strain the liquid over fresh ice cubes in a glass rather than serve a drink with the partially melted ones in the shaker.

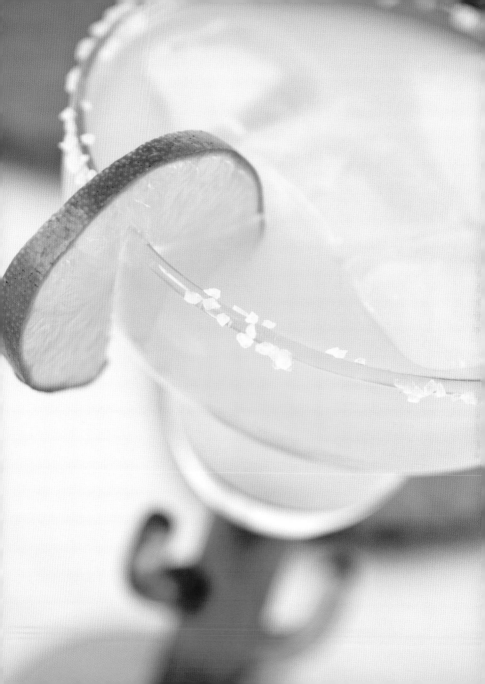

Stemware

Everything tastes better when sipped from the appropriate vessel! If you don't already have elegant stemware, this could be a great time to indulge. A beautiful glass gives the Preggatini a sexier feel in your hand, and it will continue to be treasured post-pregnancy. This list of stemware corresponds to the simplistic way I've described the glasses in drink recipes throughout the book (the definitions in a traditional bar manual may vary slightly).

BAR MUG: Thick, heat-resistant glass mug typically used to insulate cold or hot drinks

CHAMPAGNE FLUTE: Tall, narrow champagne glass

CHAMPAGNE SAUCER: Round, bowl-shaped champagne glass

COCKTAIL GLASS: Any smallish, pretty piece of stemware not otherwise defined in this list

MARGARITA GLASS: Very wide-rimmed, bowl-shaped glass used especially for margaritas

MARTINI GLASS: Tall, thin-stemmed glass with a V-shaped bowl

ROCKS GLASS: Short, stout glass

SHOT GLASS: Small glass, typically measuring about one ounce of liquid

TALL GLASS: Tall, cylindrical glass used for mixed drinks; often called a Collins glass in "bar speak"

WINE GLASS: Stemware with a smaller, narrower bowl typically used for white wine

WINE GOBLET: Stemware with a wider, rounder bowl typically used for red wine

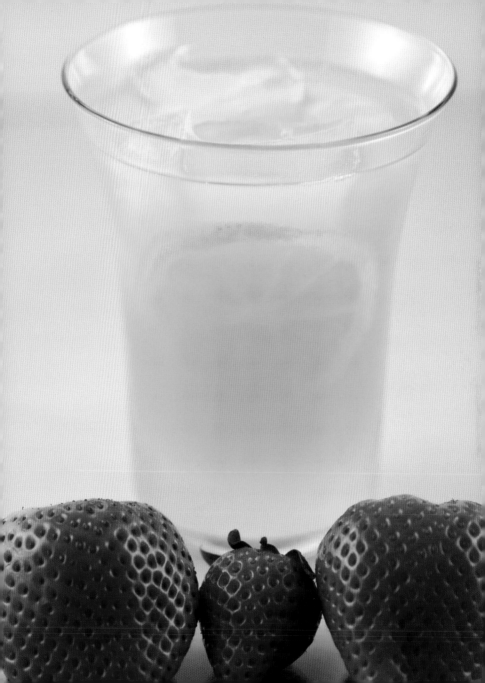

Kitchen Appliances

The term *bar chef* is becoming popular in today's high-end bars, with good reason. Many skilled bartenders and mixologists who are passionate about creating a quality experience in a glass actually spend time in the kitchen preparing their own syrups, purees, and other culinary enhancements. The drinks in this book largely reflect the bar chef philosophy, so many of your basic kitchen appliances will be useful in your Preggatini home bar, too!

BLENDER: Necessary for smoothie-style drinks

FOOD PROCESSOR: Makes crushing ice, grinding dry goods, or pureeing fruits and vegetables quick and easy

JUICER: Freshly juiced fruits and vegetables, rather than frozen or bottled, make a big difference

SAUCEPANS: Needed for stove-top preparations

Ingredients for Preggatini Fun!

If you've ever had a sickly sweet "martini" drink that gave you an instant sugar rush (and subsequent headache), chances are that it wasn't made from fresh, natural ingredients and balanced to incorporate a full flavor profile. In addition to sweet sensations, it is important to include a little citrus, a dash of cream, or even fresh herbs, spices, or other condiments to create an exciting and unique beverage. These are some ingredients to keep on hand so you can whip up your favorite Preggatini whenever a craving strikes!

ACCESSORIES: Umbrellas, swizzle sticks, cocktail picks, coasters, flavored rimming sugar, colored straws

BITTERS: Heralded for their medicinal qualities, bitters have been used to settle minor gastric ailments for over two centuries. They are made by brewing herbs, roots, and/or bark in alcohol. Using bitters is like using extract in a cookie recipe: Only a couple of drops are added, and there is a range of flavors on the market. If the alcohol in bitters concerns you, check with your doctor before using them, and consider them an optional ingredient throughout this book. (One great alternative is Stirrings Blood Orange nonalcoholic bitters; see the Cosmompolitan Cooler recipe, for example.)

DAIRY: Milk, whipping cream, half-and-half

EXOTIC INGREDIENTS: Coconut milk, coconut water, tamarind nectar, açaí juice, lychees, Thai chilis, jalapeños, rose water

FRESH FRUIT, JUICES, AND NECTARS (BUY FRESH AS NEEDED, USE FROZEN WHEN OUT OF SEASON): Lemons, limes, blood oranges, grapefruit, pineapple, watermelon, cantaloupe, honeydew, mangoes, peaches, raspberries, blueberries, blackberries, cherries, pomegranates, guava, apricots

FRESH HERBS (BUY AS NEEDED): Basil, dill, rosemary, cilantro

FRESH VEGGIES (BUY AS NEEDED): Tomatoes, cucumbers, celery, carrots, beets

GARNISHES: Rimming sugar, lavender, rose petals, edible flowers, maraschino cherries

MIXERS: Club soda, ginger ale, ginger beer (it's nonalcoholic), tonic water, flavored waters, flavored organic Italian spritzers

QUALITY ICE: Ice is as much an ingredient as anything else that goes into a good cocktail. Large, solid cubes melt slowly (so they don't water down the drink) and don't break into slivers in the cocktail shaker. Invest in a few ice cube trays with deep cavities, and use purified water for the best-tasting drinks. Also, experiment with ice cubes made with juices and mixers— as they melt, the drink becomes more flavorful!

> To get a great drink, start with quality ingredients.
>
> "You can't build a Ferrari out of Ford parts."
>
> —Tony Abou-Ganim, founder of TheModernMixologist.com and author/host of *Making Great Cocktails at Home*

SIMPLE SYRUP (SEE RECIPE ON FACING PAGE): This is essentially sugar water cooked into a syrup. It is used for sweetening cocktails because the sugar is already dissolved and won't leave granules in the drink.

SPICES AND CONDIMENTS: Fresh ginger, black pepper, cayenne pepper, Worcestershire sauce, horseradish, agave honey, Tabasco, sugar, cloves, cinnamon sticks, nutmeg

SIMPLE SYRUP

2 cups sugar (use raw, organic, white sugar as a healthier option)

1 cup water

Pour sugar and water into a small saucepan, stirring constantly. Allow mixture to come to a boil, then reduce heat to low and let simmer for 5 minutes, stirring occasionally. Cool and refrigerate in glass jar or plastic bottle. For a slightly different taste, use raw brown sugar instead of white.

Variations

Ginger-infused simple syrup: Add a 1-inch piece of peeled ginger to the saucepan, and follow simple syrup directions.

Chili-infused simple syrup: Add one Thai chili to the saucepan, and follow simple syrup directions.

Rose-infused simple syrup: Follow simple syrup directions, but use rose water instead of plain water. (Potable rose water can be found in specialty stores and Middle Eastern markets.)

🍸 The Liquid Muse Mixology Tip:
Blend plain simple syrup and fresh lemon juice (to taste) instead of using bottled sweet-n-sour. You won't want premixed after you try fresh!

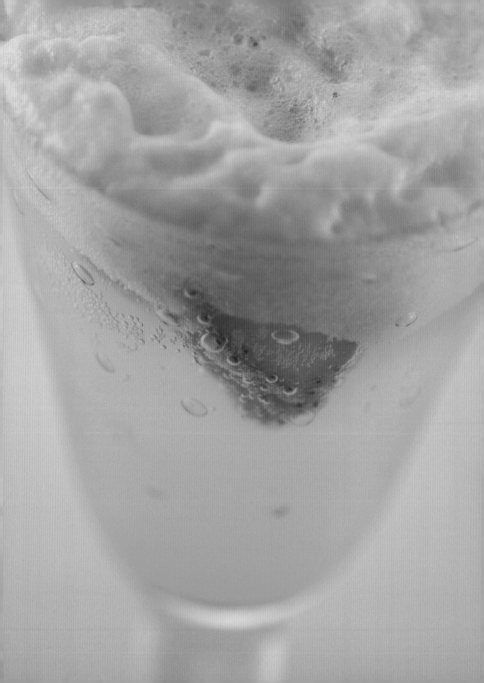

Part 2

"DE-VIRGINIZE" FOR DADS (AND OTHERS)

The main focus of this book is on the mom-to-be. However, there is someone else expecting a baby: the daddy! Some men give "support through solidarity" and lay off the sauce while their ladies can't indulge, which is a thoughtful (and rare) show of team spirit. However, the best way to say "I empathize" might be as simple as grabbing a cocktail shaker and serving as the designated master Preggatini-tender. The "De-Virginize" instructions sprinkled throughout this book were created with these wonderful dads-to-be in mind, so they can whip up a tasty concoction for both of you with a little added "kick" in theirs.

The following rules of thumb allow *Preggatinis* to remain a useful cocktail book long after the doctor says it is safe to drink alcohol again. Don't be afraid to experiment. As I teach in The Liquid Muse Cocktail Classes, there are no right or wrong answers when it comes to your own favorite drink. With or without alcohol, cocktails are fun!

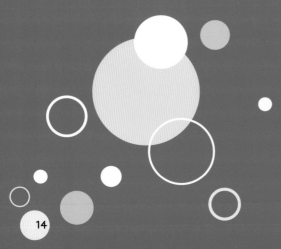

When in doubt, use vodka. An ounce or two of vodka will not change the taste of the drink too much and is a safe bet when you want to add a spirited kick. That being said . . .

Don't discount gin. Vodka has replaced gin in too many modern versions of classic cocktails. Even the beloved martini was originally created with gin. You owe it to yourself to experiment with the flavor profile of the myriad of botanicals infused into a quality gin.

Tequila is your friend. If your only exposure to tequila was in shots and "poppers" during spring break, you have not experienced the sophisticated side of the spirit of Mexico. A fine sipping tequila rivals the smoothness of a high-end cognac and makes for a wonderful cocktail.

Tropical juices beg for rum! Create variety by using spiced rum, dark rum, or light rum. Each brings its own characteristics to a drink. Class it up by exploring artisanal "rhums" from boutique distilleries throughout the Caribbean.

Creamy drinks go well with brandy. Go high brow by adding an ounce of aged cognac for sophisticated flare.

Make friends with foreigners. Look beyond your comfort zone and play with spirits that traverse global borders, such as Chilean/Peruvian pisco, Brazilian cachaça, Japanese sake, Korean soju, French eau de vies, and the recently re-legalized absinthe used in classic pre-Prohibition cocktail recipes.

Substitute orange-flavored liqueur for orange juice. You can keep the orange juice in the drink, if desired, or leave it out and use an ounce of orange-flavored liqueur.

Substitute champagne for club soda. In many of the drinks topped with club soda or nonalcoholic sparkling wine, champagne will do nicely.

Use more than one. Get creative by adding an ounce of a base spirit (e.g., tequila, vodka, gin, whisky, etc.) and a half-ounce of an additional liqueur. Apple, ginger, raspberry, elderflower, coffee, and anise are only a few flavor options in high-quality liqueurs.

"Cocktails are sexy and play a leading role in the perfect courtship. Now the wedding is a distant but sweet memory and a new chapter is beginning in your lives: She is pregnant. It is a great feeling, the beginning of your family; so much lies ahead. Then Saturday night rolls around and you decide to stay at home and cook, cozy up in the nest. He makes himself a dry martini, and then it hits . . . what does she drink? Approach nonalcoholic cocktails with the same attention given their stronger cousins. Use good glassware and fresh ingredients, and garnish with style."

—Dale DeGroff, President of the Museum of the American Cocktail, and author of *The Craft of the Cocktail*

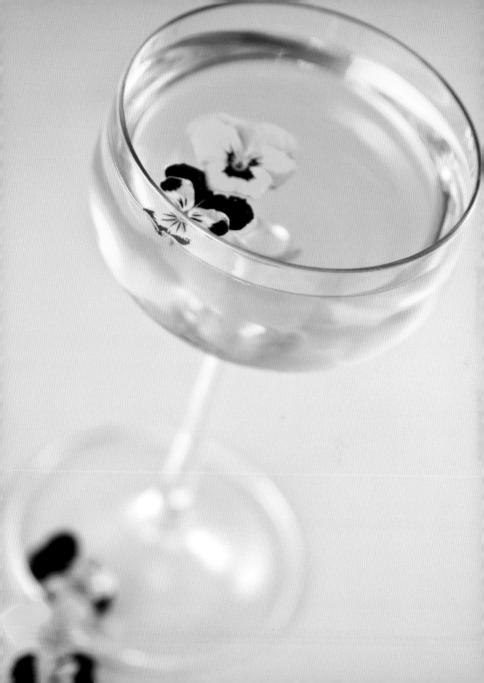

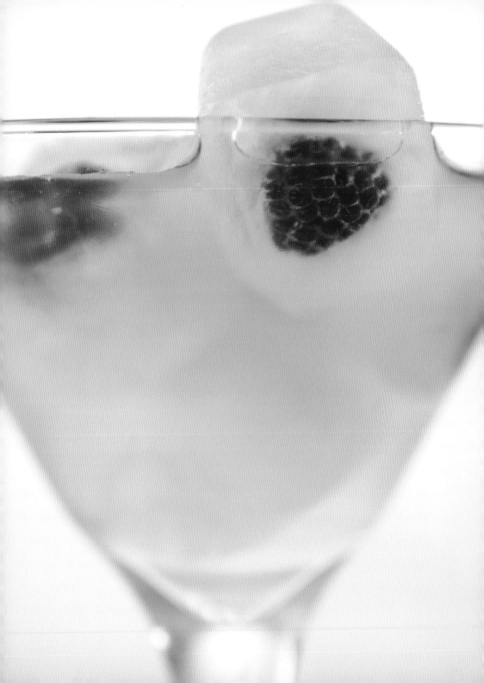

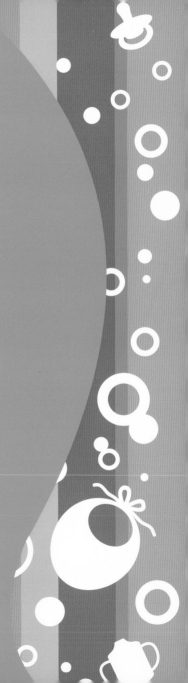

Part 3
THE RECIPES

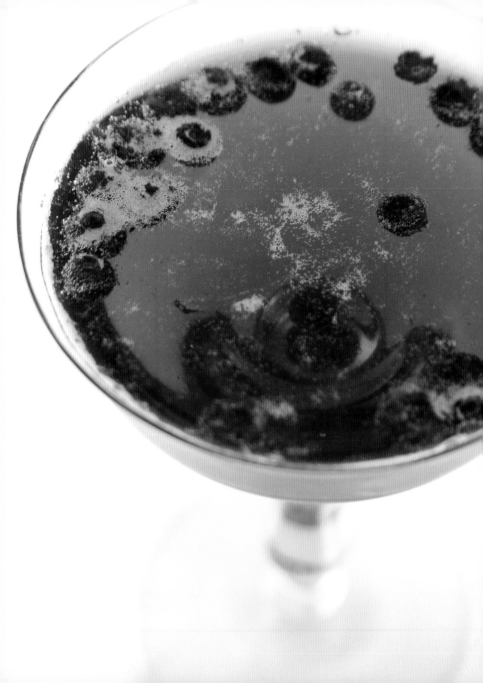

1

PRE-PREGNANCY: PROCREATE

Some women go to extremes when it comes to alcohol before conception. They pile on the partying before a long, dry year ahead and then make an abrupt 180-degree turn, tossing their wine glasses out the window. Although you will swear off alcohol pretty soon, this transition can be less dramatic—and drinking Preggatinis ensures that you can continue to enjoy that fancy stemware you got for your wedding!

Want to live it up with a few "final fling" cocktails, cool down your wild streak by detoxifying from the inside out, and then set things on fire in the bedroom? This chapter shows you how, starting with a few of The Liquid Muse Signature Cocktails to enhance your last-chance tippling. When you're serious about incubating a fetus and ready for a little internal spring cleaning, move on to the "detox" Preggatinis. And finally, when it's time to get down to the business of getting down, seal the deal by plying your man (and yourself) with liquorless liquid aphrodisiacs. You can even (try to) contain your excitement with Anticipation, the last drink in this chapter. A soothing sipper, designed to quell your nerves while you await those home pregnancy test results.

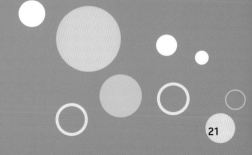

The Last Hurrah

For the party girls who want to "go big" before they "go bust" for the next three-quarters of a year, here's an invitation to The Liquid Muse cocktail party! Take a good look. This may be the last liquor you'll be sipping for a while.

 BOUQUET OF ROSÉ
(Champagne Saucer)

When Napa's Domaine Carneros (Taittinger Champagne) launched its sparkling Brut Rosé, it did so with a Signature Cocktail designed by The Liquid Muse. I took my cue from light fruit aromas inherent to the bubbly and added some subtle enhancement, swirled with a hint of romance.

Spritz rose water

½ ounce rose-infused simple syrup

3½ ounces sparkling rosé

Sprig fresh lavender

Spritz a chilled champagne saucer with rose water. Pour in rose-infused simple syrup (recipe page 11) and sparkling rosé. Lay a sprig of fresh lavender across the top of the glass as an aromatic garnish.

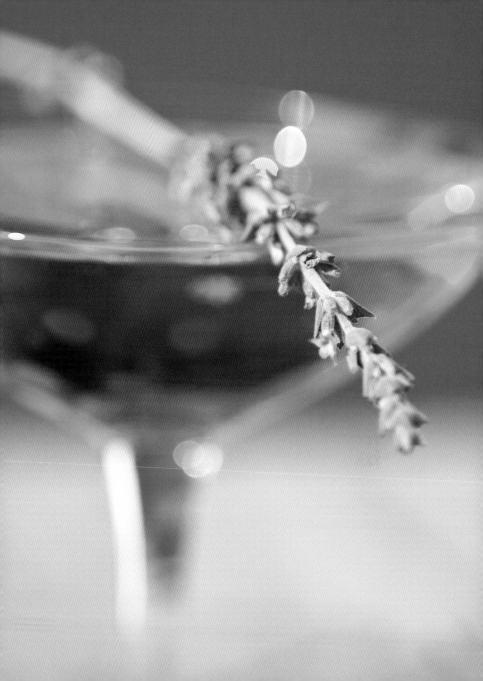

TRUMP THIS!
(Martini Glass)

Yes, Donald Trump seems to own one of everything—including his own vodka brand! When Trump Vodka asked me to design a cocktail for the product Web site, my aim was to make something unusual and exotic . . . in other words, a drink for the person who already has everything (except a baby bump, of course).

1½ ounces Trump vodka

1½ ounces tamarind nectar (can be found in ethnic supermarkets)

1 ounce coconut milk

½ ounce lime juice

1 teaspoon freshly grated nutmeg

Shake vodka, tamarind nectar, coconut milk, and lime juice with ice. Strain into a chilled martini glass. Top with freshly grated nutmeg.

> "Drinking just to get drunk is like having sex just to get pregnant."
>
> **—Robert Hess, renowned mixologist and editor of DrinkBoy.com**

QUEEN OF HEARTS
(Martini Glass)

Watching reality shows such as The Girls Next Door *is one of my guilty pleasures. So, I was extra-excited when hired to create four poker-themed cocktail recipes for the 2007 Celebrity Poker Tournament held at the Playboy Mansion. (Figuring out what to wear was a different story entirely!) This drink is very girly—pink, sweet, and creamy: perfect for the pre-pregnancy days . . . and nights.*

Granulated sugar

1½ ounces vodka

1 ounce white chocolate liqueur

1 ounce cream (or half-and-half)

½ ounce maraschino syrup

1 maraschino cherry

Rim a martini glass with granulated sugar and set aside. Pour all liquid ingredients into a mixing glass, then cover and shake well with ice. Gently strain into the rimmed glass, and finally drop the maraschino cherry into the bottom of the glass.

BILLION-AYRE'S BET
(Rocks Glass)

When the popular gambling site Bodog (www.bodoglife.com) enlisted my services to design an exclusive Signature Cocktail for its handsome billionaire bachelor CEO, Calvin Ayre, I created a refreshing accompaniment to his breezy, glamorous lifestyle.

3 ounces Bombay Sapphire gin

2 ounces freshly squeezed grapefruit juice

Squeeze of lime

¾ ounce Campari

A splash of champagne

1 lime wheel

Shake gin, juices, and Campari with ice cubes. Strain and pour into a rocks glass filled with fresh ice cubes. Top with champagne. Garnish with a lime wheel.

> *Campari is an Italian liqueur infused with herbs, spices, and fruit rinds. Created by Gaspare Campari in the 19th century, this classic spirit is refreshing when mixed with club soda and ice on hot summer afternoons or served as an aperitif before dinner on a balmy evening.*

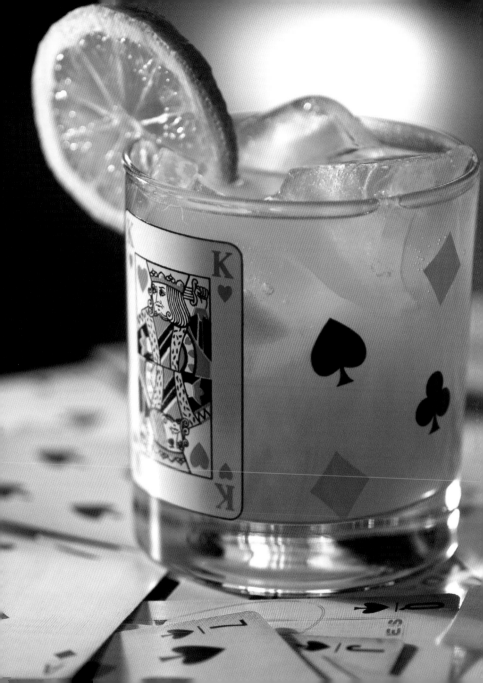

Cleaning House

I hope you got a good eyeful of tempting cocktail recipes, because now we are moving on to the serious task of having a whole lot of fun with liquorless libations! Before bringing a baby into the world, and into your body, there is a little prep work to be done. Flush out toxins with plenty of water, and start taking those prenatal vitamins. It's time to put prudence before partying and treat your body like the temple it is so it's prepared for a nice, long visit from you-know-who!

CLEAN LIVER
(Bar Mug)

Everything we eat—and drink—gets filtered through the liver. Milk thistle, the crucial ingredient of this warm tonic, is thought to aid in detoxifying the liver, while mint helps sooth digestive ailments.

1 milk thistle tea bag*

3 sprigs fresh mint

1 teaspoon wildflower honey

1 lemon wedge

Pour boiling water over the tea bag and fresh mint, and let steep for 3–5 minutes in a bar mug. Remove tea bag and mint, and stir in the honey until it dissolves. Garnish with a lemon wedge.

*If you may already be pregnant, double-check all herbal remedies with your doctor before ingesting.

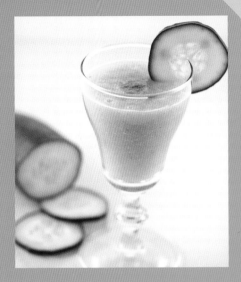

 INSIDE SPA
(Cocktail Glass)

Have you ever had cool, soothing cucumber slices placed on your eyes during a facial? Or sipped cucumber water while waiting for a massage at a spa? This refreshing cucumber concoction aims to hydrate your baby-making organs from the inside out, while the cayenne pepper is believed to stimulate internal cleansing.

- ½ cucumber, peeled, seeded, and diced
- ½ ounce lemon juice
- 1 teaspoon sugar
- 1 ounce sparkling water
- Pinch ground cayenne pepper

Put diced cucumber into a food processor. Add lemon juice and sugar and blend on low for 1 minute. Pour mixture into a large, ice-filled cocktail glass. Top with sparkling water and sprinkle with a pinch of ground cayenne pepper.

De-Virginize for Dad :
Add 1½ ounces Square One organic cucumber vodka or Hendricks gin, which both have hints of cucumber flavor.

POMEGRANATE COOLER
(Tall Glass)

Pomegranates are packed with vitamin C, niacin, and iron. (They have even been declared a "super fruit" by the media, including Oprah Winfrey, who is said to be fond of pomegranate martinis.) Blueberries and grapes are also full of antioxidants, making this cooler a one-two punch!

5–7 fresh or frozen blueberries

3 ounces pomegranate juice

2 ounces white grape juice

3 ounces sparkling pomegranate soda

1 lemon slice

Muddle the blueberries in the bottom of a tall glass. Then add ice and pour in the juices. Fill the glass to the top with sparkling pomegranate soda, and place a lemon slice on top of the drink. Sip through a colorful straw.

De-Virginize for Dad 🍸**:** Along with the juices, add 1 ounce vodka and ½ ounce PAMA pomegranate liqueur.

> 🍷 *According to Greek lore, Persephone (the sunny-dispositioned daughter of Zeus) is forced to spend four months each year in the underworld because she could not resist the temptation of eating seeds from a forbidden pomegranate. During her absence the earth becomes cold and barren— in other words, this is the Ancient Greek explanation for winter.*

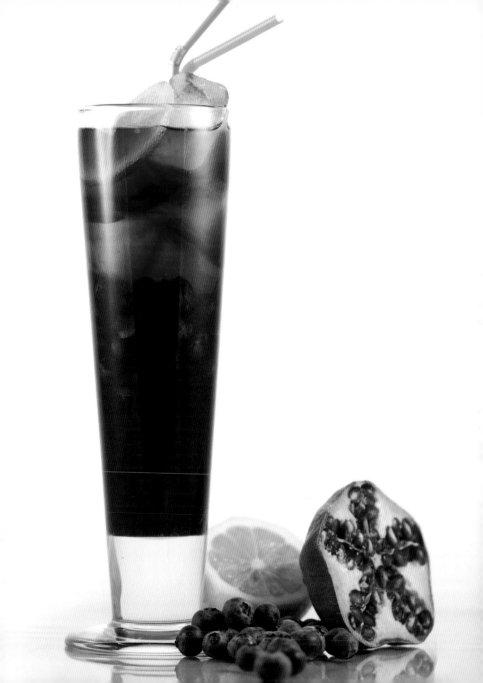

Getting Down to Business

Ok, so your body is not only a temple—it's also a pleasure palace! Some would argue that the best part of being pregnant is getting pregnant. This next round of non-boozy-floozie drinks is designed to keep you—and your man—up to the task of baby-making. Drawing from a range of so-called aphrodisiacs, these Preggatinis help get the real party started. Brew some passion potions in your cauldron of seduction so when ovulation strikes, you can enjoy a delicious nonalcoholic drink and have a darn good time in the process!

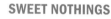

SWEET NOTHINGS
(Champagne Flute)

If your guy is the romantic type, this cocktail may set the stage for a soiree d'amour. Remember, you can spike his with real sparkling wine if you think he may need a little encouragement.

½ ounce freshly squeezed lemon juice

1½ ounces tangerine juice

1 ounce mango juice

3 ounces nonalcoholic sparkling wine

¼ ounce grenadine

1 maraschino cherry

Pour juices into a champagne flute. Gently add the nonalcoholic sparkling wine. Slowly pour in the grenadine, which will sink to the bottom of the glass. Garnish with a maraschino cherry, and test your guy's talents by seeing if he can tie the stem in a knot with his tongue.

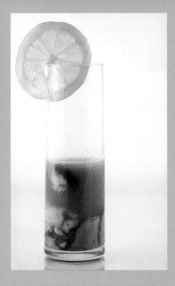

■ OYSTER SHOT
(Shot Glass)

If you've ever been on a hot date at a seafood restaurant, you may remember a gleam in the fella's eye as he ordered a dozen oysters for an appetizer. Long rumored to be a mouthful of hot lovin', oysters are high in zinc, which boosts progesterone levels, directly affecting the libido.

1 plump, juicy oyster, shucked*

¼ ounce lemon juice

½ ounce tomato juice

Dash Worcestershire sauce

¼ teaspoon horseradish

Place the oyster in a shot glass. Pour in all liquids and top with the horseradish (another spicy kick). Shoot it down all at once.

*If you may already be pregnant, check with your doctor before eating raw seafood.

De-Virginize for Dad
: Add 1 ounce chilled premium vodka with the other liquids.

PANTS ON FIRE
(Martini Glass)

Ignite a night of hot passion by sipping a nonalcoholic cocktail with a kick! This spicy tipple includes lust-inducing chili and passion fruit, which is said to have a calming effect. Perfect for a relaxing-yet-exciting night in.

1 ounce passion fruit puree

3 ounces pineapple juice

1 ounce guava nectar

1 ounce chili-infused simple syrup

1 ounce prickly pear syrup (or grenadine)

1 Thai chili

Pour passion fruit puree, juices, and chili-infused syrup (recipe page 11) into a mixing glass. Shake with ice. Strain into a chilled martini glass. Gently pour prickly pear syrup into the drink, allowing it to settle at the bottom of the glass. Garnish with a Thai chili on a toothpick on the side of the glass.

De-Virginize for Dad ➤ : Place 3 or 4 Thai chilis in his favorite bottle of vodka. Let sit for at least one week. The spirit will have absorbed flavor and spice from the pods—and it will keep getting hotter over time! Shake 1 ounce of the fiery vodka along with the juices and simple syrup.

> ● *Spicy foods act as an aphrodisiac and are even said to rev up the metabolism. So get the party started—and keep it going—with chili!*

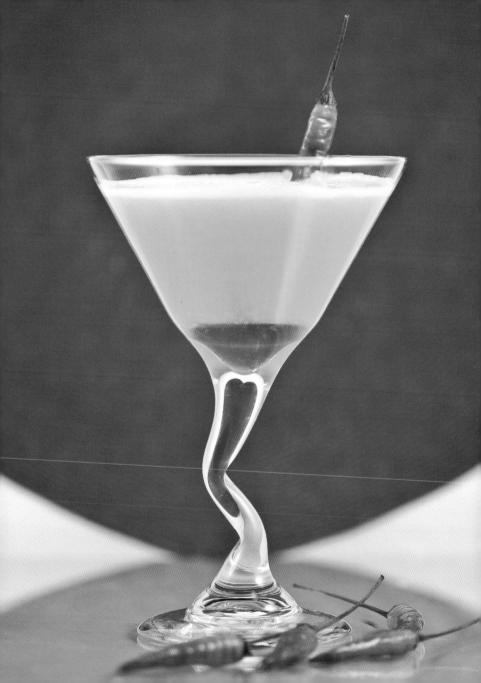

Drum Roll, Please

After all that hard work, it's time for the moment of truth. Did you conceive, or are you sentenced to another month of hot sex with your man? (If you're not in a hurry to get pregnant, this could be a winning situation however you look at it.) No matter what the result, taking a pregnancy test can be a nerve-wracking experience, so here's a drink to sooth your anxieties.

ANTICIPATION
(Cocktail Glass)

You bought the box. You completed the awkward task of wetting the stick. Now you wait. It may be only a few minutes, but it can feel like forever. Here's something to keep your mind, and your taste buds, occupied.

4 ounces chamomile tea

1 teaspoon wildflower honey

½ ounce lemon juice

1 edible flower

Brew a cup of chamomile tea, and let it cool to room temperature. Pour 4 ounces of tea into a mixing glass. Add the wildflower honey, and stir until dissolved. Add the lemon juice, and fill the mixing glass with ice. Shake, then strain into a chilled cocktail glass. Garnish with an edible flower.

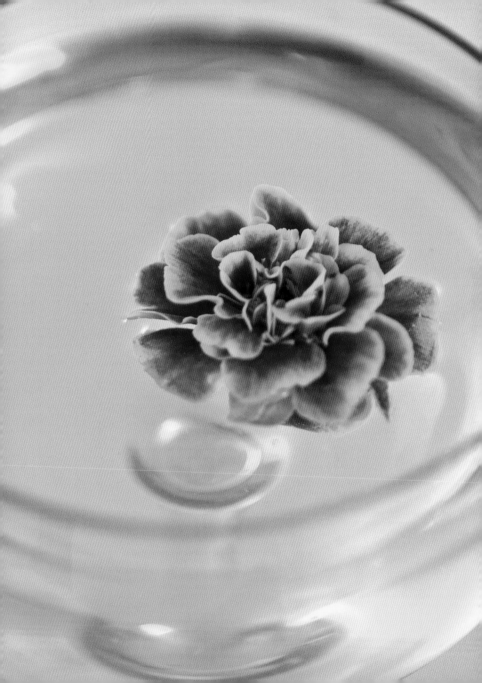

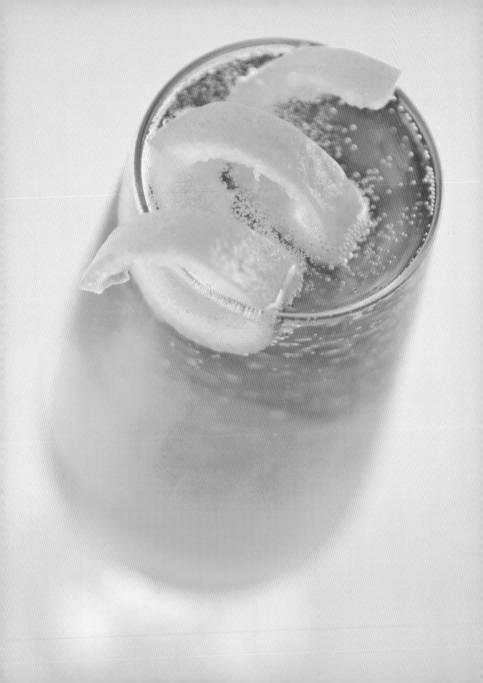

2

FIRST TRIMESTER: GERMINATE

Congratulations, you got knocked up! Whether this is your first baby or your fifth, a long-cherished dream or a (gulp) wonderful surprise, your egg and his sperm can rightfully declare "Mission Accomplished." It's time to celebrate your ability to procreate.

In our modern world, women become mothers in a whole rainbow of scenarios: In addition to the traditional boy-meets-girl, boy-marries-girl, boy-gets-girl-pregnant-and-they-all-live-happily-ever-after script, some women fly solo into motherhood with their planned, or unplanned, bundles of joy. Whatever your circumstance, you're about to welcome a baby into a loving home, the threshold of which is your uterus!

It is important to take extra special care of you because your body is now your baby's temple. Even though *you* may be puking up your decaf lattes these first few months of pregnancy, it is important to try to incorporate extra nutrients into your diet. This chapter addresses worshipping yourself, and your thriving reproductive system, as the fertile goddess you are!

The first section offers drinks for a little celebration à deux; then come a slew of Preggatinis centered around ginger, which is believed to ease queasiness (and thus morning sickness). Last, I've concocted several fanciful drinks filled with folic acid, which is integral to fetal development during the first trimester.

Impregnation Celebration

Nothing says "Whoopee!" like a special drink to punctuate the occasion. These recipes are designed to enhance the private celebration between you and whomever you hold dearest. Here's to a job well done!

THREE'S COMPANY
(Tall Glass)

A baby transforms a couple into a family. It is a living, breathing expression of the love you have for your partner and deepens already profound bonds. In other words, this third wheel is a welcome addition.

3 thinly sliced lemon wheels

3 ounces pink lemonade

3 ounces bitter lemon soda

3 strawberries

Fill a tall glass with ice. Line the glass with lemon slices. Pour in pink lemonade and lemon soda. Garnish with three strawberries on a cocktail skewer laid across the top of the glass.

De-Virginize for Dad 🍸: Add 1 ounce citrus-flavored vodka and ½ ounce limoncello, a sweet Italian lemon liqueur.

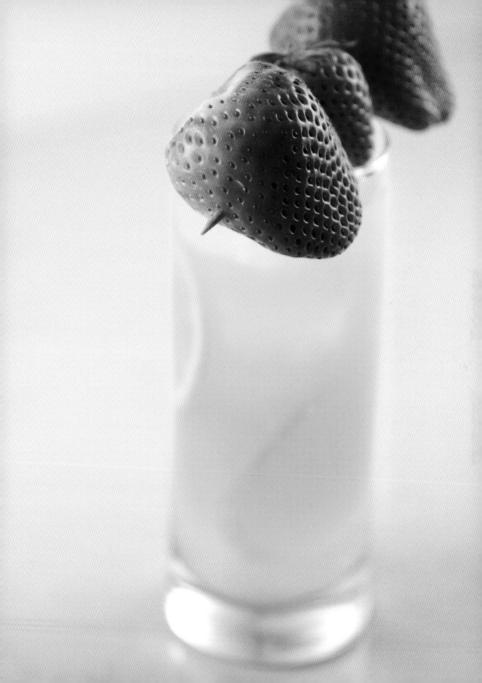

DRINKING FOR TWO
(Champagne Saucer)

While some things in life remain ambiguous (Are white shoes after Labor Day no longer a fashion faux pas?) there is no doubt what a "plus" sign indicates on your home pregnancy test. Any way you read it, this is a done deal and you're now eating—and drinking—for two.

1 slice jalapeño

1 teaspoon orange marmalade

½ ounce lemon juice

1 ounce orange juice

3 ounces nonalcoholic sparkling wine

Muddle jalapeño slice with marmalade and lemon juice in the bottom of a mixing glass. Add orange juice and ice, then shake vigorously. Strain into a champagne saucer. Add the nonalcoholic sparkling wine.

> ☞ *Did you know that cocktail glasses originally held only 4 or 5 ounces of liquid? That's about half the size of what is used in today's bars, many of which serve 8- to 12-ounce martinis. (No wonder we wake up with pounding heads!)*

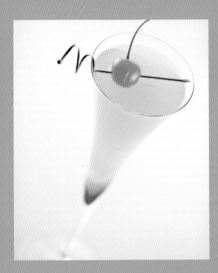

BABY ON BOARD!
(Champagne Flute)

For the next nine months, wherever you go, so goes baby. Your tummy is a taxi whose passenger has settled in for the ride of a lifetime. Instinct makes you extra cautious of every move you make, so isn't it fun to know that drinking Preggatinis while hauling this cargo isn't hazardous in the least? (Now go get one of those little triangular signs for your car!)

2½ ounces mango nectar

1 ounce lime juice

2 ounces lime-flavored sparkling water

1 maraschino cherry

Pour mango nectar, lime juice, and sparkling water into a champagne flute. Garnish with a maraschino cherry on the edge of the glass.

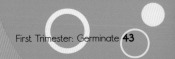

The Morning After
(and After, and After . . .)

Normally, if you woke up feeling queasy after all that celebrating, I'd suggest that you down a gallon of water, take an aspirin, and have a nice, long nap until the alcohol worked itself out of your system. However, as much as I hate to bring it up, you may be worshipping the porcelain god for a couple of months—and it has nothing to do with liquor! The next round of drinks is built around ginger, nature's answer to an upset tummy and morning sickness.

APRICOT GINGERINI
(Martini Glass)

This Preggatini mingles the soft flavor of apricot with sweetened ginger and gentle white grape juice, which is by itself a recommended beverage during the first weeks of pregnancy. Additionally, this drink includes a dash of ground clove—another ancient remedy for pregnant ladies experiencing nausea.

2½ ounces white grape juice

3 ounces apricot nectar

1 ounce ginger-infused simple syrup

¼ teaspoon ground clove

Pour grape juice, apricot nectar, ginger-infused simple syrup (recipe page 11), and most of the ground clove into a mixing glass filled with ice. Shake vigorously, then strain into a martini glass. Garnish with the remaining ground clove atop the drink.

De-Virginize for Dad : Reduce the grape juice by 1½ ounces, then add 1 ounce gin and ½ ounce ginger liqueur.

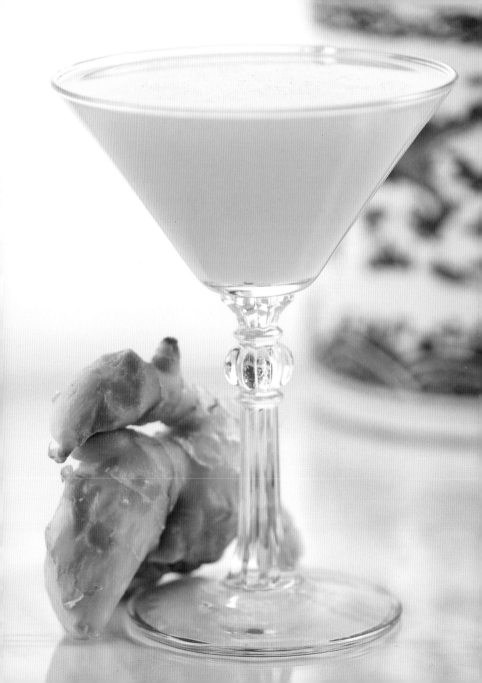

GINGERLY GESTATING

(Bar Mug)

Warm and soothe a troubled tummy with this ginger tea drink. In addition to smelling wonderful, mint is also helpful in reducing an "icky" tummy. If you're pregnant during summer, this Preggatini can be served over ice. This recipe makes two servings.

Small bunch fresh mint

**1 heaping tablespoon freshly grated ginger
(or 1 organic ginger tea bag)**

1 teaspoon lavender or wildflower honey

Pour two cups of boiling water over mint and ginger (or tea bag) in a teapot. Let steep 5 minutes. Stir in honey until dissolved. Pour into bar mugs or teacups.

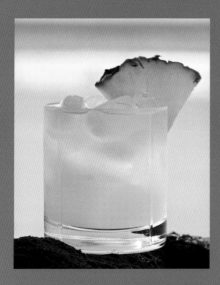

PREGGIE PARADISE
(Rocks Glass)

Dreaming about meeting your baby-to-be and preparing for his or her arrival is one of the happiest times of your life, despite any temporary queasiness! Lift a glass to the little one.

2 ounces pineapple juice
Dash Stirrings Blood Orange bitters
3 ounces ginger beer
1 pineapple wedge

Pour the juice, bitters, and ginger beer into a rocks glass filled with ice. Garnish with a pineapple wedge on the edge of the glass.

De-Virginize for Dad : Reduce ginger beer by 1 ounce, and add 1½ ounces rum.

Frolicking with Folic Acid

Folic acid, also known as folate, is one of the building blocks of life and an integral nutrient during the first few months of pregnancy. By now you're taking prenatal vitamins, which are meant to supplement folate, calcium, and iron during this crucial time in your baby's early development. The following drinks support that effort with ingredients such as cantaloupe, kiwi, strawberries, blackberries, papaya, spinach, and beets.

FOLIC FIZZ
(Wine Glass)

Cantaloupe's folic quotient makes it among the best choices for First Trimester Preggatinis. This one is punctuated with iron-rich strawberries to make it extra tasty and good for you!

½ cup cantaloupe chunks

3 large strawberries

½ ounce lime juice

1 ounce simple syrup

Lime-flavored mineral water

Put the cantaloupe through a fruit juicer, then pour 3 ounces of the resulting juice into a wine glass. Slice 2 strawberries and put them into the glass. Add the lime juice and simple syrup, then add ice and stir gently. Top with lime-flavored mineral water, and garnish with the remaining strawberry on a cocktail pick.

De-Virginize for Dad : Add 1 ounce ginger liqueur along with the juices and top with champagne instead of mineral water.

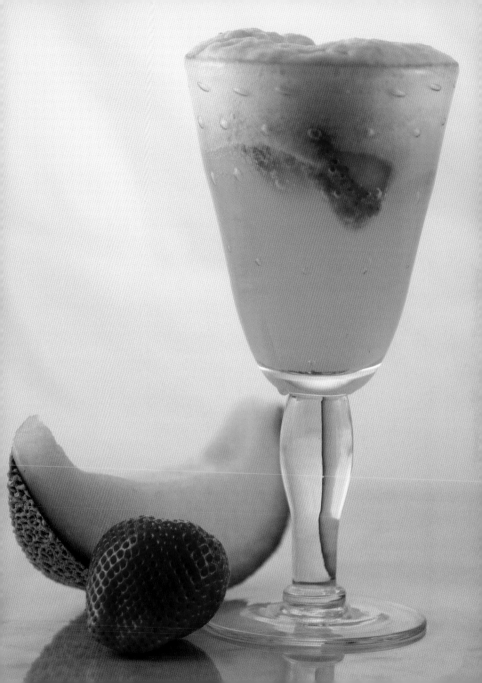

GLASS OF GLOW
(Cocktail Glass)

Are people already starting to mention how radiant you look? In addition to hormonal surges, your glow comes from taking better care of yourself! Just consider pregnancy nature's way of making you even more beautiful.

3 ripe blackberries

½ ounce simple syrup

½ ounce lemon juice

3 ounces Glow Mama kiwi drink* or kiwi juice

1½ ounces club soda

1 slice kiwi

Gently muddle the blackberries, simple syrup, and lemon juice in the bottom of a cocktail glass. Add ice, then pour in Glow Mama and club soda. Garnish with a slice of kiwi on the side of the glass.

*Available online and in select maternity stores and natural food stores

FRUITY FOLATE SHAKE
(Tall Glass)

Papayas are loaded with folate, and bananas are high in potassium. Add a swirl of sweet coconut milk, and this blended Preggatini is a great boost of energy any time of the day.

½ cup fresh papaya chunks (or ⅓ cup papaya nectar)

½ banana

1 ounce coconut milk

4 ice cubes

1 slice papaya

Pinch grated coconut

Blend first four ingredients for 30 seconds or until smooth. Pour into a tall glass. Garnish with a long slice of papaya and a sprinkle of grated coconut.

De-Virginize for Dad 🍸: Add 1 ounce coconut-flavored rum into the blender.

FEEL THE (HEART) BEET
(Rocks Glass)

By the end of the first trimester, you will hear your baby's heartbeat. This drink includes spinach—high in iron to fortify the red blood cells pulsing through your umbilical cord—as well as beets and carrots, which are full of vitamin C and folic acid. They're also high in sugar, making them as sweet as fruits.

3 carrots

½ cup spinach

½ beet

Extract juice from the veggies one at a time in a standard juicer, and pour the resulting liquid into a rocks glass. The colorful combination is pleasing to the eye as well as the palate!

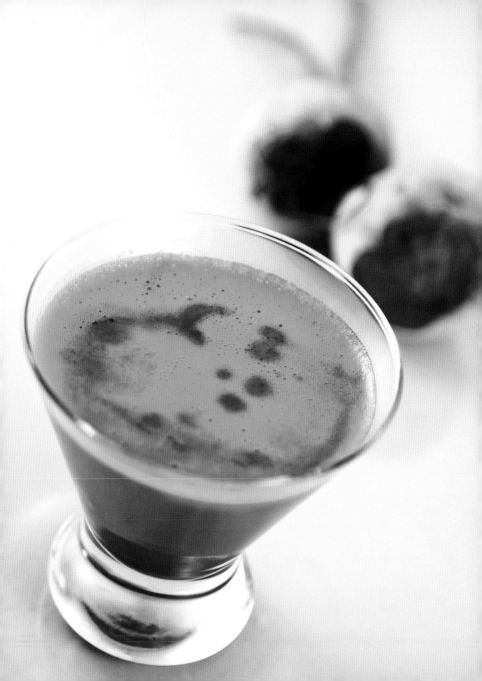

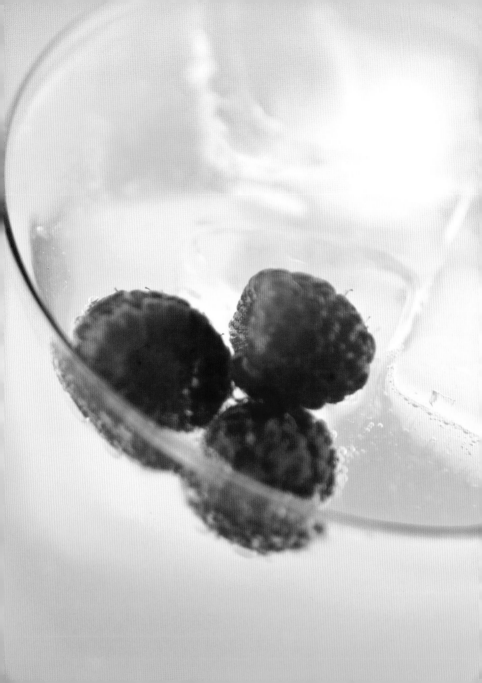

3

SECOND TRIMESTER: PROCLAMATE

Many newly pregnant moms decide to wait until the second trimester to sing their good news from the rooftops. And when they do, everyone wants to wish them well! Over the next few months, you will be the toast of your personal and professional acquaintances (sans alcohol, of course).

This book is filled with festive drink recipes to make at home . . . but what do you do when you go out? Never fear! The first section of this chapter highlights cocktail menu alternatives and tells you how to order them so any well-heeled bartender, worldwide, will know exactly what you want. I've also "virginized" a few popular cocktails for you to make at home so you don't have to live without your favorite drinkie while baby is in your belly.

The biggest celebration of this trimester may be the latest trend for parents-to-be . . . the babymoon! It's a chance to get away from the hullabaloo and stay up all night doing what got you pregnant in the first place, before you're up all night changing diapers! The Preggatinis in the third section of this chapter set the mood for that final fling, whether you're at a seaside resort or in a snowy chalet—or just snuggled up at home with the blinds down.

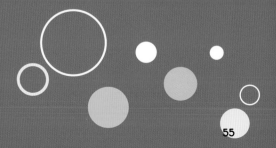

Belly Up to the Bar

As you transition from barfly to baby mama, you may wonder what to order during the next girls night out. After all, what fun is it to feel like a wallflower sipping sparkling water while all your girlfriends are clinking colorful, tasty drinks in pretty glasses? Here are some nonalcoholic cocktails you can order from any bartender and sound like a pro!

MADRAS MIA
(Tall Glass)

Order it like this: I'll have a virgin Madras with a splash of club soda and a lemon wedge.

A Madras is vodka with cranberry and orange juices. It is a basic drink that any bartender will know. Here's how to turn it into a Preggatini.

2 ounces cranberry juice

2 ounces orange juice

1 ounce club soda

1 lemon wedge

Pour all liquid ingredients into a tall glass filled with ice. Garnish with a lemon wedge on the rim of the glass.

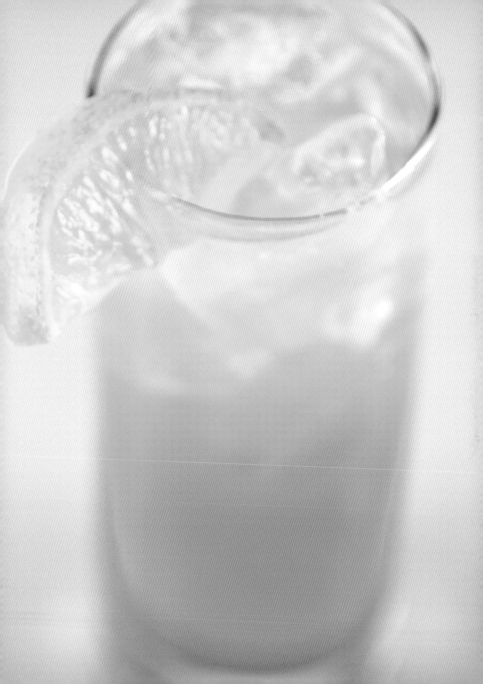

SALTY PUPPY

(Martini Glass)

Order it like this: I'd like a virgin Salty Dog in a martini glass with a splash of tonic.

The time-tested Salty Dog is a common drink made with gin or vodka and grapefruit juice in a glass rimmed with salt. (Without the salt-rimmed glass, the drink is called a Greyhound.) Make it preggie-friendly by leaving out the booze and adding a little tonic water.

3 ounces grapefruit juice

1 ounce tonic water

Rim a martini glass with salt. Slowly pour in the grapefruit juice and tonic water.

> ➥ *Photograph Your Beautiful Belly. How often will you proudly expose your midsection after gaining 30 pounds? That alone is worth a party . . . and pictures! Celebrities like Demi Moore and Christina Aguilera made it mainstream to pose exposed for magazine covers in their third trimesters. Why not schedule your own belly-centric photo shoot and create a keepsake album?*

THE LIQUID MUSE EASY-PEASY PREGGATINI
(Martini Glass)

Order it like this (with a big, friendly smile): I'd like pineapple and grapefruit juice with a splash of cranberry and a squeeze of lime shaken and strained into a martini glass, topped with a splash of soda. Please.

This Preggatini is made with a delicious combination of juices available in any bar in the world. It is also easy to whip up at home, or in a friend's home, when socializing.

2 ounces pineapple juice

2 ounces grapefruit juice

½ ounce freshly squeezed lime juice

Splash cranberry juice

Splash club soda

Pour first four ingredients into an ice-filled mixing glass. Shake, then strain into a martini glass. Top with a splash of soda.

MOMOSA
(Champagne Flute)

Order it like this: Please bring my orange juice in a champagne flute. Add a splash of simple syrup, and top it with club soda.

If your favorite part of brunch is a mimosa (orange juice and champagne), this option will keep you smiling all day long. Obviously, nonalcoholic sparkling wine would be the ideal substitute; keep that in mind when making this recipe at home. However, as not all restaurants carry it, club soda and a splash of simple syrup (recipe page 11) will do the trick. If there is no simple syrup on hand, just add a teaspoon of sugar and stir.

3 ounces orange juice

1½ ounces nonalcoholic sparkling wine or club soda

½ ounce simple syrup (if using club soda)

Pour ingredients into a chilled champagne flute.

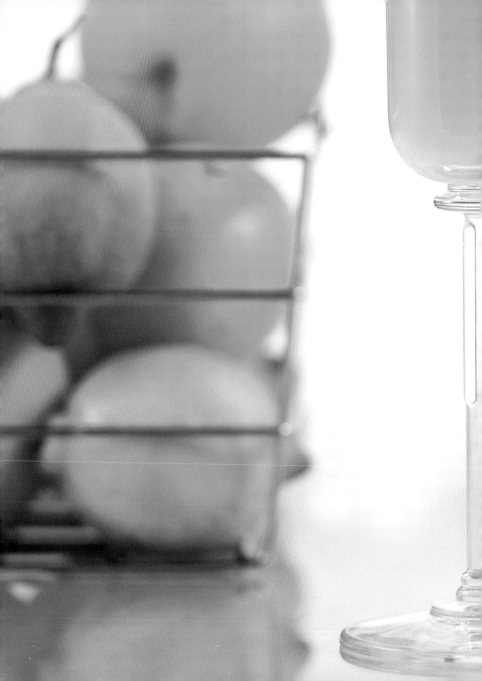

Oldies But Goodies

Even though nonalcoholic cocktails are finally beginning to catch on in restaurants, the ingredients for virginized classics may or may not be available in bars. Relax. These easy-to-follow directions give you the power to be mistress of your own liquid pleasure, even while you're drinking for two!

MAMARITA
(Margarita Glass)

Can't imagine a platter of sizzling fajitas without a margarita? This Preggatini version of your favorite Mexican concoction will have you dancing to the beat of your own mariachis!

2 tablespoons rimming salt

1 ounce agave nectar (found in health food stores)

½ ounce freshly squeezed lemon juice

1 ounce orange juice

3 ounces limeade

1 lime wedge

Salt-rim a margarita glass and set aside. Stir agave nectar and lemon juice in the bottom of a mixing glass until nectar dissolves. Add orange juice, limeade, and ice, then shake vigorously. Strain into the margarita glass, and serve with a lime wedge.

De-Virginize for Dad ➤: Turn the Mamarita into The Liquid Muse Margarita by leaving out the limeade and orange juice. Fill a cocktail shaker with ice and vigorously shake 2½ ounces tequila, ½ ounce orange-flavored liqueur, 1½ ounces lime juice, and ½ ounce agave nectar (absolutely NO bottled sweet-n-sour mix). Strain into a salt-rimmed martini glass and serve "straight up" or into a salt-rimmed margarita glass filled with fresh ice. Garnish with a lime wheel.

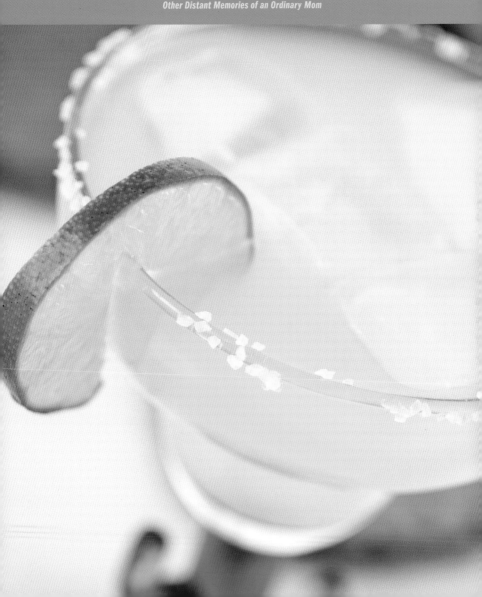

"By my second trimester, I started dreaming about my delivery. In the dream, I popped the baby out effortlessly and, immediately, the nurse handed me a big ol' margarita on the rocks, no salt. Turns out, that dream never came true. But I do remember my first post-pregnancy martini with my girlfriends at our local bar. It's the best drink I've ever had."

——Brett Paesel, author of *Mommies Who Drink: Sex, Drugs, and Other Distant Memories of an Ordinary Mom*

MAKE MINE A MOMJITO!
(Tall Glass)

If the Latin cocktail craze has hit your 'hood, then you've probably sampled a whole myriad of creative incarnations of the mojito. This one stays close to a traditional recipe—only without the rum.

1 lime, diced with peel on

5–6 mint leaves

1 teaspoon brown sugar

1 ounce Torani Butter Rum syrup

Lemon-lime soda or club soda

1 lime wheel

Muddle diced lime, mint, sugar, and syrup in the bottom of a tall glass. Fill with ice. Top with lemon-lime soda or club soda, depending on how sweet you want it. Garnish with a lime wheel.

De-Virginize for Dad ✎: Use 1½ ounces rum or cachaça (Brazilian sugarcane liquor) instead of the butter rum syrup to make this drink more like a traditional mojito or caipirinha.

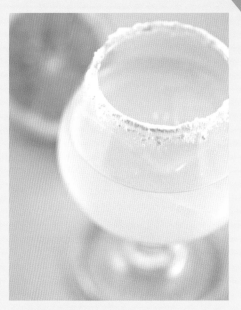

 VIRGIN LEMON DROP
(Cocktail Glass)

If your favorite drink is the sweet and tart Lemon Drop, sipping this nonalcoholic Preggatini will satisfy that tongue-tingling desire.

Powdered sugar

1 ounce white grape juice

½ ounce freshly squeezed lemon juice

3 ounces lemonade

Rim a small cocktail glass with powdered sugar and set aside. Shake juices and lemonade with ice, then gently strain into the glass.

COSMOM

(Martini Glass)

Any fashion-loving city slicker (or suburbanite) knows that the Cosmo was the "it" drink of the 1990s. Its overwhelming popularity has given it the staying power to become a modern classic and remain on drink menus a decade later. If that little ol' pink vodka martini is your drink, this Preggatini will keep you feeling sexy in any city.

3 ounces cranberry juice

1 ounce lime juice

½ ounce mandarin orange juice

½ ounce orange-flavored syrup

1 lime twirl

Shake juices and syrup with ice. Strain into a martini glass. Garnish with a lime twirl.

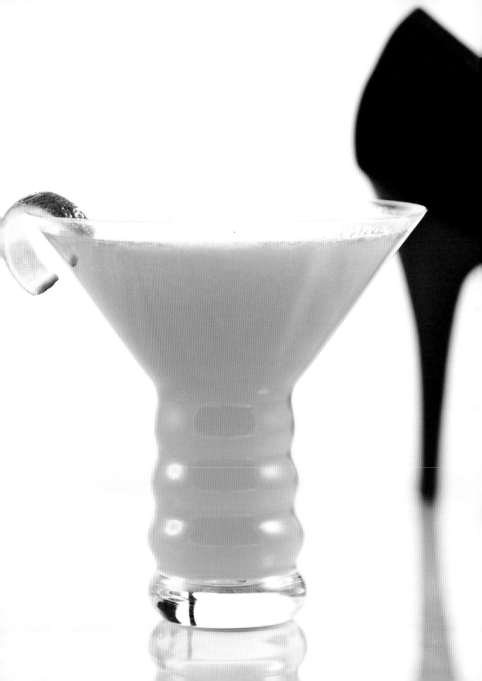

Babymoon Libations

The babymoon trend is catching on with parents-to-be who want to snag a little extra-special "us" time before baby's birth, when everyone's attention will shift to the newest member of the family. Whether your fantasy is strolling on the beach in a sunny paradise or warming each other up in a winter wonderland, these Preggatinis are designed to inspire your romantic getaway.

HAWAIIAN HIGHBALL
(Tall Glass)

You'll practically feel island breezes with every sip of this tropical treat. Slip your toes into the sand, and let exotic fruit flavors lull you into relaxation.

Stirrings Piña Colada Rimmer

3 ounces guava juice

2 ounces mango juice

1 ounce Torani Crème de Banana syrup

3 ounces club soda

Rim a tall glass with piña colada rimming sugar, then set aside. Pour juices and banana syrup into a mixing glass and shake with ice. Slowly strain into glass. Fill to the top with club soda.

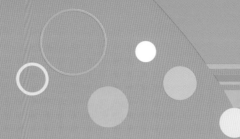

HOT BUTTERED MUM'S RUM
(Bar Mug)

This Preggatini takes off the chill on a snowy evening and is the perfect complement to buttering up your loved one in front of a roaring fire.

- **1 cup water**
- **2 whole cloves**
- **½ ounce lemon juice**
- **2 ounces Torani Butter Rum syrup**
- **1 cinnamon stick**
- **1 pat butter**

Heat water, cloves, and lemon juice in a small saucepan, then pour into a bar mug. Add butter rum syrup, and garnish with a cinnamon stick and pat of butter.

De-Virginize for Dad : Reduce the buttered rum syrup to 1 ounce, and add 1 ounce of your favorite rum.

WHITE HOT MAMA
(Bar Mug)

Most men find the mother of their unborn child even hotter than before pregnancy. Think about it: Your baby bump is proof that he is virile, and your feminine strength is taken to new heights while carrying a baby. Snuggle up and revel in the beauty of your yin and yang with this hot, creamy glass of decadence with a kick!

2 tablespoons caramel sauce

½ teaspoon ancho chili powder

½ teaspoon vanilla extract (optional)

2 tablespoons white hot chocolate cocoa powder

1 teaspoon honey

1 cup whole milk

Drizzle caramel sauce around the inside of a bar mug, particularly around the inside of the rim. Mix the remaining ingredients in a small saucepan, and bring to a vigorous simmer over medium heat. Reduce the heat to low and continue to stir for 5 more minutes. Let the mixture cool to slightly above room temperature, and gently pour into the mug.

De-Virginize for Dad : Add 1 ounce brandy and 1 ounce white chocolate liqueur to the glass before adding the hot milk mixture.

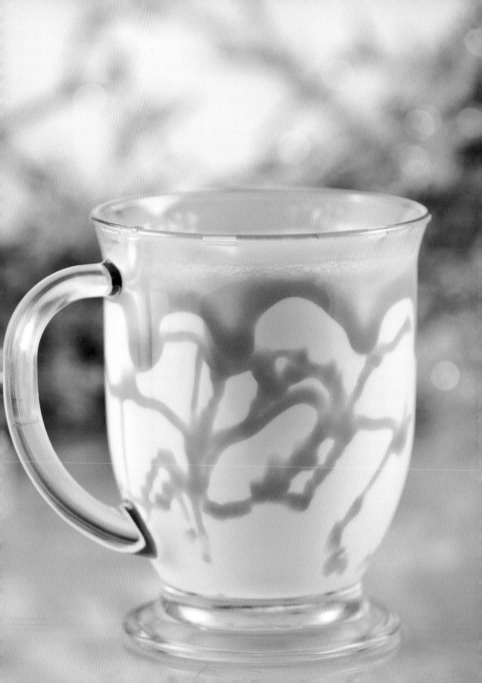

COCONUT KEY LIME MOMTINI
(Martini Glass)

Those who consider the Florida Keys the ideal getaway will love this drink's nod to the tasty, tart Key limes famously found on the American peninsula where the Atlantic meets the Caribbean.

3 ounces limeade

1 ounce coconut milk

½ teaspoon powdered sugar

1 ounce Stirrings Clarified Key Lime

2–3 drops vanilla extract (optional)

1 teaspoon coconut flakes

Shake first five ingredients with ice. Strain into a martini glass. Garnish with coconut flakes.

De-Virginize for Dad : Use only 2 ounces limeade, and add 1½ ounces coconut-flavored rum or vodka.

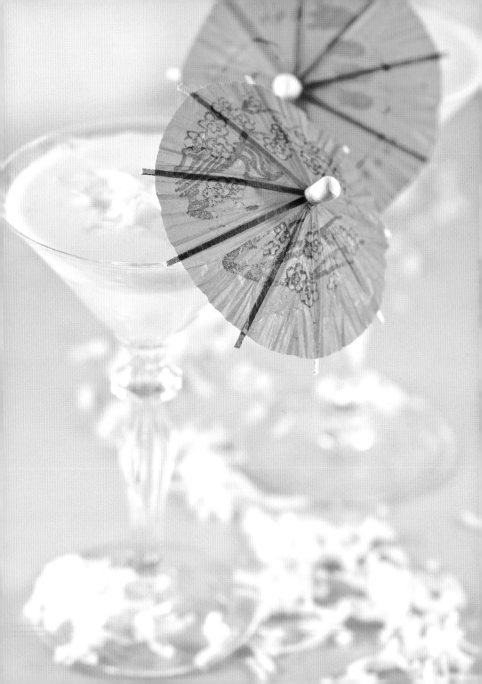

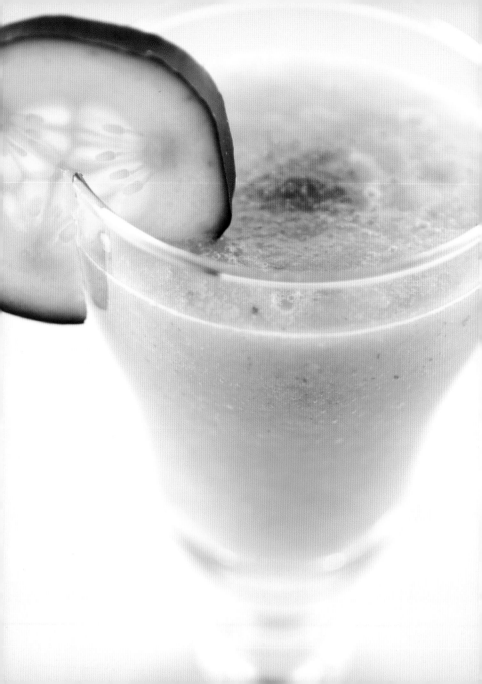

4

THIRD TRIMESTER: CULTIVATE

Living large has never been more in fashion! The bigger your baby bump becomes, the more mom-to-be "street cred" you carry. There ain't no hiding it—so use it to your advantage!

This chapter honors your special status, celebrates the little person you're about to meet, and offers some sweet relief for the last few weeks of pregnancy, which—let's face it—can be a little uncomfortable. Amid all the excitement, planning, and preparations for baby, don't forget to stop and smell the roses. You're about to be someone's mommy.

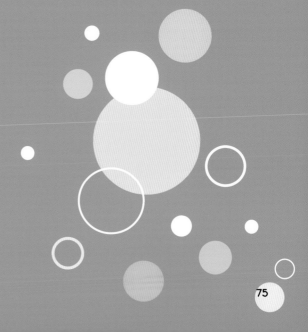

Pregnant and Proud!

Being a woman never feels more special than when you're flaunting your status as an integral link in perpetuating humanity. People offer you their seats on public transportation, hold open doors, and are only too happy to carry things for you. It's like stepping into an alternate universe filled with chivalrous knights at every turn. (Enjoy it while you can!) These drinks pay tribute to this moment in time, when every woman is entitled to a little extra-special attention.

BABY BUMP BREEZE
(Tall Glass)

Sporting a baby bump is a breeze once you're sipping a refreshing nonalcoholic cocktail created just for you. This one is also a breeze to make: Just gather a few ingredients and pour them in a glass!

2 ounces cranberry juice

3 ounces pineapple juice

2 ounces blood orange Italian soda

Pour all ingredients into a tall glass filled with ice. Garnish with a colorful swizzle stick to stir the drink.

De-Virginize for Dad : Add 1 ounce vodka or white tequila and ½ ounce VeeV açaí liqueur or PAMA pomegranate liqueur.

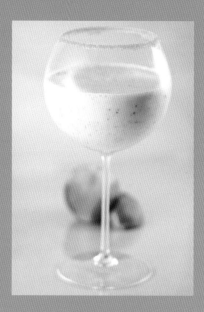

 MILFSHAKE
(Wine Goblet)

There's a reason why the terms cougar *and* MILF *have become mainstream topics of lively, even controversial, conversation. Your man may not be the only who finds you irresistible as you blossom into womanhood. More than ever, younger guys are lusting after women with more life experience. And frankly, who can blame them?*

Stirrings Bellini Rimmer

1 peach, chopped and peeled

1½ ounces apricot nectar

1 scoop vanilla ice cream

Rim a wine goblet with Bellini rimming sugar and set aside. Puree all other ingredients in a blender, and pour into the wine goblet.

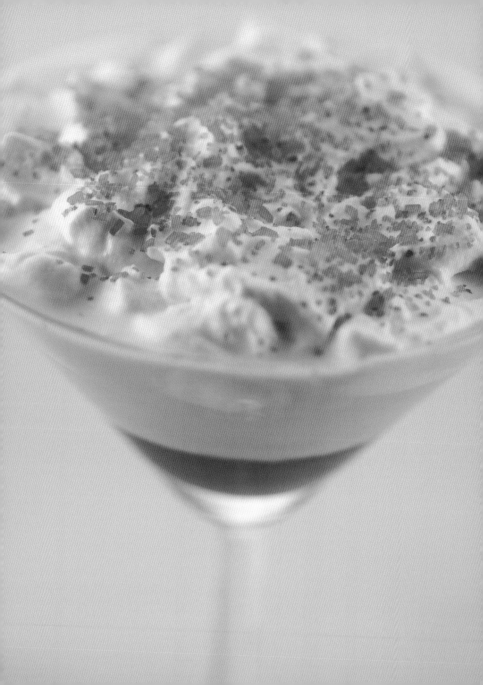

"The essence of a Hot Mom is . . . being confident and feeling empowered. Being the best mom is tied to being the best YOU. Your attitude affects and is reflected in your children—even in utero."

—Jessica Denay, founder of HotMomsClub.com and author of the
Hot Mom Handbook series

CALL ME PRINCESS PREGGATINI
(Martini Glass)

Have you ever played Queen for a Day? Well, being preggers, you get to play it every day for the better part of a year. Here's to you, Your Highness!

Granulated sugar

1½ ounces milk

1 ounce strawberry flavored syrup

½ ounce prickly pear syrup (or grenadine)

¼ cup heavy cream, lightly whipped

1 strawberry

Rim a martini glass with granulated sugar and set aside. Pour milk and strawberry syrup into a mixing glass and shake with ice. Gently add mixture to martini glass. Slowly drizzle in the prickly pear syrup or grenadine, allowing it to sink to the bottom. Spoon on the lightly whipped (slightly soupy) cream so that it becomes the top layer. Garnish with a strawberry, and serve alongside a rhinestone-encrusted tiara.

Hello in There!

Although you may have had a preference toward a daughter or a son, once your sonogram reveals who is kicking around inside your belly, you won't be able to imagine him or her any other way. For those of you who skip the surprise factor to start decorating the nursery and picking names, here are some options for you!

SWEET-N-SASSY
(Martini Glass)

Someday your adorable little angel will hit her teen years and become your biggest challenge. Driving, boyfriends, hormones on overdrive . . . there will be plenty of reasons to pace the floor at night later in her life. Be thankful for these first few months when you pace the floor with her safely in your arms.

Powdered sugar

3 ounces white cranberry juice

1 ounce lemon juice

1 ounce raspberry syrup

3 raspberries

Rim a martini glass with powdered sugar and set aside. Pour juices and raspberry syrup into a mixing glass and shake. Strain into the martini glass, and garnish with raspberries on a skewer.

De-Virginize for Dad ➤**:** Use ½ ounce Chambord raspberry-flavored liqueur instead of raspberry syrup, and add 1 ounce gin or vodka.

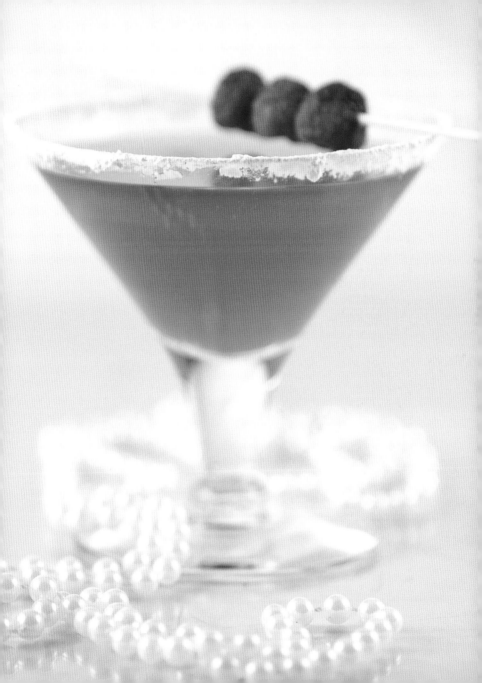

DOUBLE TROUBLE
(Cocktail Glass)

Sometimes when couples decide to start a family, they get lucky and conceive right away. And sometimes they get more than they bargained for! The first ingredient in this Preggatini is loaded with seven antioxidant-rich fruits to help you store up all the vitality you can!

3 ounces Purple antioxidant drink or pomegranate–açaí juice blend

½ ounce lemon juice

1½ ounces organic Italian black cherry spritzer

Pour Purple (or pomegranate–açaí blend) and lemon juice into a mixing glass. Add ice and shake vigorously. Strain into a cocktail glass, and top with black cherry spritzer.

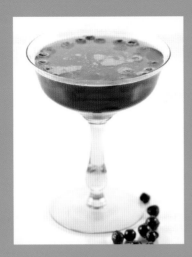

♛ LITTLE BOY BLUE
(Champagne Saucer)

If you're out of practice when it comes to nursery rhymes, it may be time to reacquaint yourself with those little ditties that make tiny tots coo. "Little Boy Blue" is a staple among baby's first forays into literature, and this drink may become a regular among your forays into Preggatinis.

> **3 ounces blueberry pomegranate juice**
> **½ ounce lemon juice**
> **½ ounce simple syrup**
> **2 ounces blueberry spritzer, preferably organic**
> **3 blueberries**

Pour all liquid ingredients into a champagne saucer. Garnish with three blueberries on a skewer across the rim of the glass.

De-Virginize for Dad ☜: Use only 2 ounces pomegranate juice, and add 1 ounce blueberry-flavored vodka. Sparkling wine can be substituted for blueberry spritzer.

Easy Does It

The closer you get to the arrival of your little one, the more ready you may become to get your body back to yourself! By the end of this trimester, you may have trouble sleeping, get a little clogged up, have bizarre cravings, or just feel slightly off balance. These Preggatinis are intended to help ease physical discomforts as the big moment draws near.

 SLEEPING BEAUTY
(Bar Mug)

Remember when your mom gave you warm milk to help you sleep when you were a little girl? Soothe yourself with this comforting bedtime remedy.

Stirrings Egg Nog Rimmer

¾ cup whole milk

2 teaspoons honey

**½ teaspoon ground cinnamon, saving one pinch
    to garnish the drink**

Rim a bar mug with egg nog rimmer. Heat all ingredients in a small saucepan, and let simmer for 5 minutes on low heat. Pour into a bar mug. Sprinkle with a pinch of ground cinnamon.

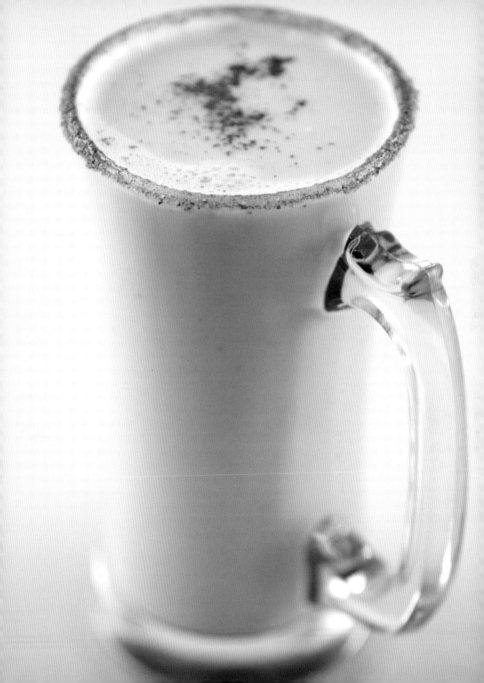

RELEASE ME
(Wine Glass)

With all that is happening inside you, it isn't uncommon to find yourself a bit "congested." This Preggatini should help get things moving in the right direction again.

3 fresh purple figs

1 tablespoon lavender honey

3 ounces prune juice

3 ounces soy milk

Omitting one fig, blend until smooth all ingredients in an electric blender. If you don't have a blender handy, muddle two figs and honey in the bottom of a mixing glass. Add prune juice, soy milk, and ice, then shake vigorously for 30 seconds. Strain into an ice-filled wine glass and garnish with the third fig on a cocktail skewer.

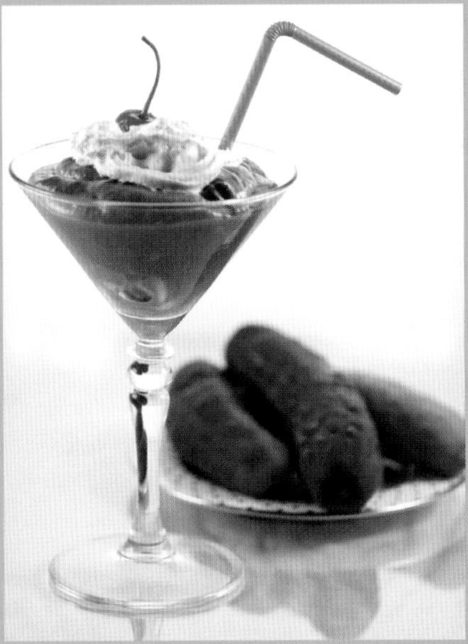

FUNKY MONKEY

(Martini Glass)

The old cliché about begging for pickles and ice cream while pregnant may not be too far off base! Here is something to satisfy you should a case of the odd cravings suddenly arise.

1 scoop chocolate ice cream

½ banana

1 tablespoon peanut butter

¼ cup milk

1 or 2 pickles

Place all ingredients in a blender and mix until smooth. Pour into a cocktail or martini glass. Serve with a side of pickles.

And Finally . . .

This Preggatini encourages you to take a moment for yourself in the weeks leading up to meeting the love of your life . . . your child.

GARDEN ROSE
(Cocktail Glass)

Hopefully you've had a chance to sit with yourself during this precious time and think about what motherhood means to you. As your belly unfurls into full bloom, budding within you is the beautiful, sacred, fragile gift of life.

1 heaping tablespoon diced cucumber (peeled and seeded)

1 ounce rose-infused simple syrup

3 ounces Fre Chardonnay alcohol-removed wine

Splash club soda

1 rose petal

Gently muddle cucumber and rose-infused syrup (recipe page 11) in the bottom of a mixing glass. Add ice and wine, then shake well and strain into a cocktail glass. Top with club soda. Garnish with a rose petal.

De-Virginize for Dad : Substitute the alcohol-removed wine with 3 ounces of your favorite Chardonnay to make a wine cocktail, or use Hendrick's gin, which has hints of rose and cucumber flavor, for a martini-style drink.

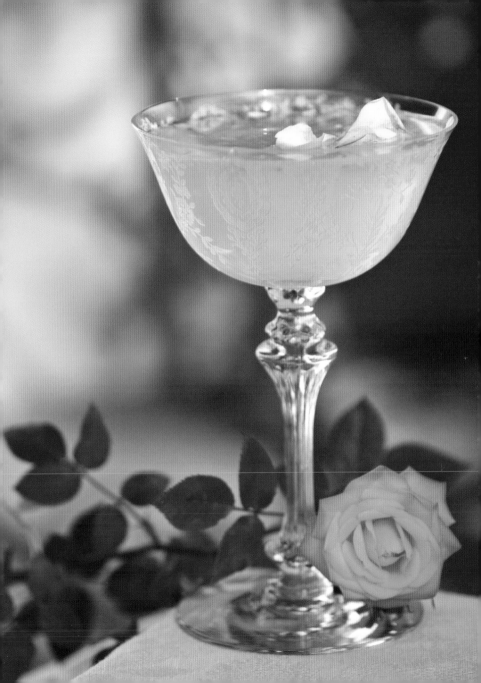

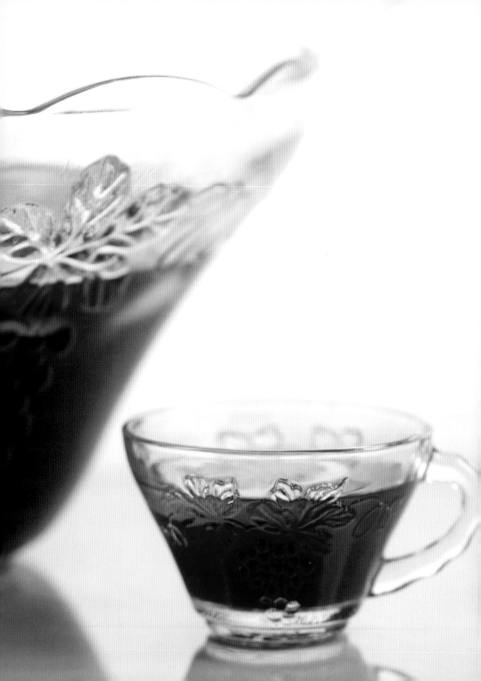

5

THE PREGGATINI PARTY™: COMMEMORATE

Customized to fit the personality of the future-mama, a Preggatini Party is the spiffed-up, modernized version of the same old run-of-the-mill baby shower. Nonalcoholic cocktails for the guest of honor bring a hip vibe to the time-treasured gathering of family and friends, turning it into one of the most talked-about social events of the year!

This chapter presents two Preggatini Party themes and drinks to go with them. Each theme includes some party suggestions of fun things to do, as well as an elegant party dip recipe from a famous chef to enhance your tippling. Be sure to also peruse the Preggatini Punches section so you can prepare larger quantities of liquid refreshments ahead of time.

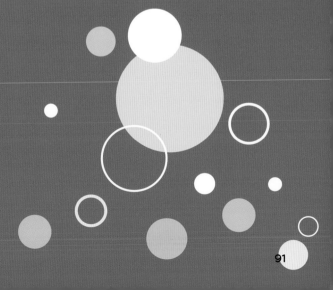

Party Like a Rock Star with CelebriBaby Preggatinis

With practically every celebrity in Tinseltown sporting a baby bump and/or toddler on the hip, it seems that "mommy" is the dream role for leading ladies and puts a song in the hearts of pop princesses. Now that you've become a member of the child-bearing jet set, toast the star in your life (your baby) with a CelebriBaby Preggatini.

KINGSTON KRUSH
(Cocktail Glass)

Ska/pop star and designer diva Gwen Stefani and her hunky hubby Gavin Rossdale rock more than the music studio, as proven by their expanding family. With a new baby stealing the spotlight, this drink was created in honor of big brother Kingston, one of the coolest little kiddos in the public eye.

> **3 ounces coconut water (or 2 ounces coconut milk)**
>
> **2 ounces açaí juice (or pomegranate juice)**
>
> **½ ounce ginger-infused simple syrup (see recipe page 11)**
>
> **¼ ounce lime juice**
>
> **½ teaspoon coconut flakes**

Pour all liquid ingredients into a mixing glass, shake with ice, then strain into a cocktail glass. Sprinkle with coconut flakes.

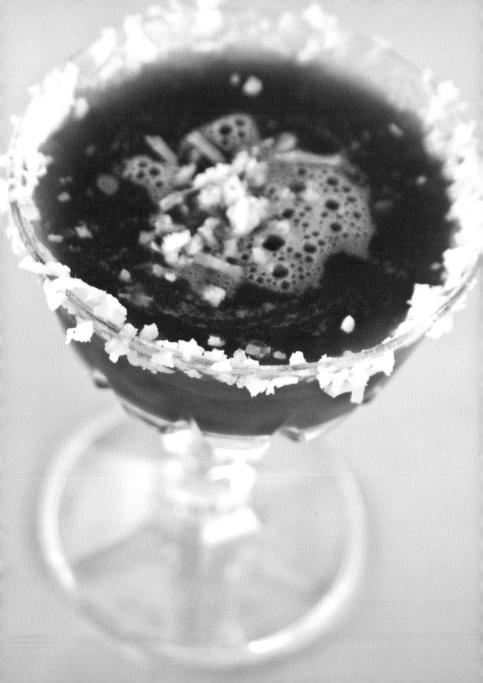

MIAMI MOMMY MOJITO

(Tall Glass)

Jennifer Lopez may have waited to start a family, but once she did it, she went big! As if she weren't busy enough running her multifaceted one-woman empire, the Latina diva (who has a history of twins in her family) took on two new full-time commitments! This Momjito is a delectable nontraditional variation that will get you swiveling your hips like a Puerto Rican princess.

1 heaping tablespoon diced strawberries

1 tablespoon torn basil

1 lime, cut into small chunks with peel on

4 ounces Fre White Zinfandel alcohol-removed wine

Splash lemon-lime soda

Muddle strawberries, basil, and lime in the bottom of a tall glass. Add ice. Fill with alcohol-removed white zinfandel, and finish with a splash of lemon-lime soda.

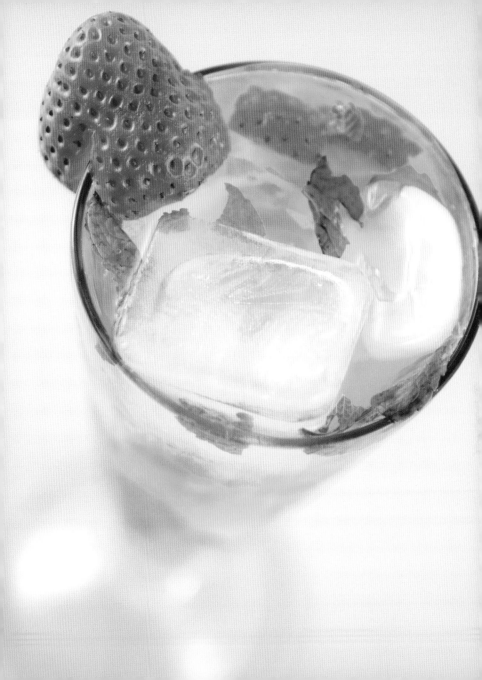

APPLE MARTIN-I
(Martini Glass)

There are many reasons to envy beautiful, Oscar-winning Gwyneth Paltrow, but one of the biggest is her sensitive-yet-sexy hubby, Coldplay front man Chris Martin. Though naming their firstborn Apple raised a few eyebrows, the moniker is an irresistible inspiration for a Preggatini.

1 tablespoon caramel sauce

3 ounces apple cider

½ ounce lemon juice

½ ounce Fee Brothers Spiced Cordial syrup

2 ounces sparkling apple cider

3 slices dehydrated apple

Drizzle caramel sauce in a swirling motion around the inside of the martini glass and set aside. Pour cider, lemon juice, and cordial syrup into a mixing glass, then shake with ice. Strain into the caramel-swirled glass, and top with sparkling apple cider. Garnish with slices of dehydrated apple on a cocktail skewer.

BERRY CHERRY BLOSSOM
(Martini Glass)

Prior to giving birth to a gorgeous daughter with her supermodel boyfriend, Gabriel Aubry, the stunning Oscar-, Emmy-, and Golden Globe–winning actress Halle Berry said that she would consider adopting a child if she didn't have one biologically. Happily for her, and the rest of us mere mortals, two of the most beautiful people on the planet mated. This drink celebrates their contribution to future "Top 10 Most Beautiful People" lists everywhere.

3 blueberries

3 raspberries

3 pitted Bing cherries

½ ounce lemon juice

½ ounce simple syrup

3 ounces cherry juice

2 ounces organic Italian black cherry spritzer

1 edible flower

Gently muddle blueberries, raspberries, cherries, lemon juice, and simple syrup (recipe page 11) in the bottom of a cocktail shaker. Add cherry juice and ice. Shake and strain into a martini glass. Top with black cherry Italian spritzer, and garnish with an edible flower floating on the surface of the drink.

De-Virginize for Dad ✎: Replace half the cherry juice with 1½ ounces EFFEN black cherry vodka.

FLOSSY AUSSIE
(Martini Glass)

Australian A-lister Nicole Kidman made no secret of her baby longings. Already the doting mother of two gorgeous kids adopted with her ex, the classic beauty and her hubby, Aussie country rocker Keith Urban, were thrilled to announce the arrival of baby Sunday. This CelebriBaby Preggatini includes a neighborly nod to New Zealand with its kiwi embellishments.

3 kumquats, halved with peel on

¼ kiwi, diced with skin on

½ ounce lime juice

½ ounce simple syrup

3 ounces Glow Mama kiwi drink*, or kiwi juice

2 ounces bitter lemon soda

Skewer of kiwi and kumquats

Muddle kumquats, diced kiwi, lime juice, and simple syrup (recipe page 11) in the bottom of a mixing glass. Add kiwi drink and shake with ice. Strain into a martini glass, and top with bitter lemon soda. Garnish with a fruit skewer on the rim of the glass.

*Available online and in select maternity stores and natural food stores

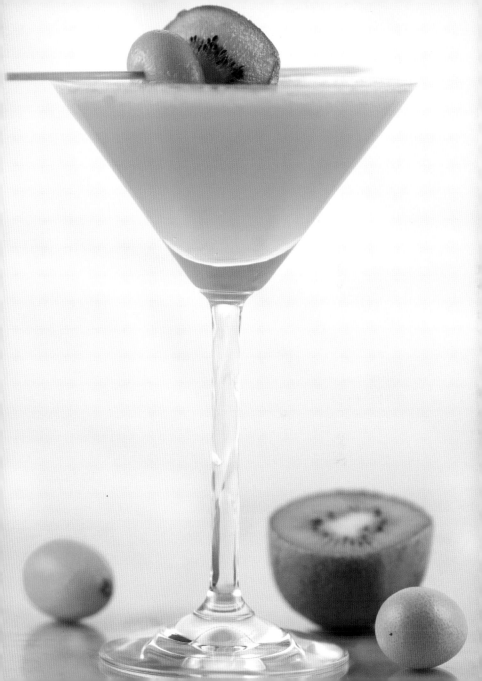

MR. MOM
(Rocks Glass)

Dads may not get enough credit for playing the supporting role during this special time. If you decide to share the spotlight and throw a coed Preggatini Party, this boozy libation draws from classic inspiration to give the papa-to-be a manly, and fully leaded, drink.

1½ ounces rye whiskey

1 teaspoon powdered sugar

½ ounce lemon juice

Dash bitters

Splash club soda

1 lemon wedge

Pour whiskey, sugar, lemon juice, and bitters into a mixing glass. Shake, then strain into a rocks glass filled with fresh ice. Add a splash of club soda, and garnish with a lemon wedge.

YELLOW TOMATO PARTY DIP WITH GRUYERE CHIPS (Serves 6–8)

From the kitchen of celebrity chef Michel Richard. Printed with permission.

DIP

1½ pounds large yellow tomatoes

1½ tablespoons finely minced shallots

1 garlic clove

1 teaspoon Dijon mustard

½ teaspoon soy sauce

¼ teaspoon granulated sugar

1 teaspoon drained capers, chopped

1 teaspoon minced chives

1 teaspoon extra virgin olive oil

Fine sea salt and freshly ground black pepper, to taste

Tabasco sauce, to taste

Preheat oven to 250°F. Cut out the cores from the tomatoes, then cut each tomato in half, lengthwise. Place cut side up on a parchment-lined baking sheet, and slowly roast them for 3 hours. Meanwhile, bring a small pan of water to a boil. Add the shallots and blanch quickly, just until tender. Drain in a fine-mesh sieve and run cold water over them to cool. Drain on a paper towel. Remove the tomatoes from the oven. Discard the skins and scoop out the seedy centers. Chop the tomato flesh and place in the center of a cheesecloth and wring out the excess liquid. Place the tomatoes in a medium bowl, add the shallots, and grate the garlic directly on top. Mix in the remaining ingredients, and refrigerate until cold (at least 1 hour). Check the seasoning again before serving.

GRUYERE CHIPS

8 very thin slices of Gruyere (ask the deli to slice it for you)

2 tablespoons chopped chives

Preheat oven to 250°F. Line a baking sheet with a Silpat (nonstick baking mat) and arrange cheese slices upon it, leaving about 2 inches between them. Sprinkle with chopped chives. Bake for about 15 minutes, until the cheese has melted and become golden brown. Remove from oven and let the chips firm up on the pan. When they are easy to remove, lift them with a spatula and place on paper towels or parchment paper to cool completely. Use the Gruyere chips to scoop up the dip, and *mange*.

> "Friends are here to enjoy life with you. Present them with the food that you love. For example, although I'm French, I stay away from heavy pâtés. I love to serve dips and refreshing, easy-to-eat cold hors d'oeuvres in shot glasses . . . mini beet salad, beans, cold soups. Also, if you serve a special dish, print the recipe for your friends and let them take it home! Be creative, modern, have fun."
>
> —Michel Richard, recipient of the James Beard Foundation 2007 Outstanding Chef Award, author of *Happy in the Kitchen*, and creator of gourmet fare at Citronelle and Central in Washington, D.C., and at Citrus at Social in Hollywood.

Zen Out

If you would rather chill out than whoop it up, this Preggatini Party theme might be more your speed. These recipes have a bit of Far Eastern flare to complement the mom-to-be who practices relatively clean and peaceful living even when not with child.

YOGI-TEANI
(Wine Glass)

If you're the kind of person who needs her daily dose of Downward Dog and greets each day with a Sun Salutation, then this tea-based Preggatini will help you stay connected to your inner yogi.

4 ounces Yogi Tea brand Woman's Mother to Be, room temperature

1 teaspoon raw brown sugar

Raspberry-lemonade ice cubes*

Pour tea and sugar into a mixing glass, and shake well with ice. Strain into a wine glass. Drop in 2 or 3 raspberry-lemonade ice cubes.

*Raspberry-Lemonade Ice Cubes

2 cups lemonade

Approximately 14 raspberries

Fill ice cube tray with lemonade. Place 1 raspberry in each cube. Freeze.

♈ The Liquid Muse Mixology Tip: *Getting creative with ice cubes brings extra flare to a drink. Freeze lemonade, exotic juices, or even tonic water for extra flavor, color, and pizzazz.*

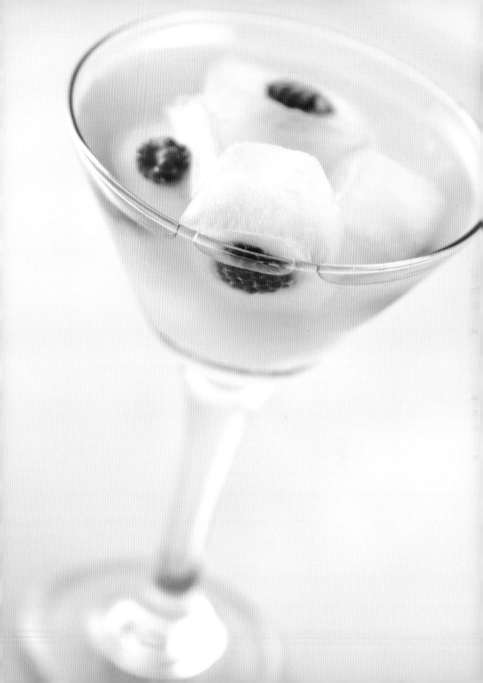

SPARKLING JASMINE BLOSSOM
(Champagne Flute)

White tea is naturally so pure that it undergoes very little process-
ing. It is believed to be even more healthful than green tea. This
Preggatini's subtle flavors will lull you into a sublime state of con-
tentment.

4 ounces organic white jasmine tea, chilled

1 ounce tangerine juice

Splash club soda

½ teaspoon freshly grated ginger

Pour tea and juice into a champagne flute. Top with club soda.
Sprinkle ginger on top.

Zen Out Preggatini Party Suggestions

☞ *Hire a massage therapist to give each guest a stress-relieving
10-minute back, neck, and shoulders rub.*

☞ *Either by following a book or by bringing in a professional,
feng shui the baby's nursery to ensure positive energy and good
luck as soon as the little one arrives home.*

☞ *Relieve the expectant mom's aching back or swollen ankles
with a gift certificate to an acupuncturist.*

MEDITERRANEAN LAYER DIP WITH TOASTED PITA TRIANGLES

From The Most Decadent Diet Ever!
© *Devin Alexander. Reprinted with permission.*

- **1 cup garlic-flavored hummus**
- **½ cup fat-free plain yogurt**
- **¼ teaspoon ground cumin**
- **½ teaspoon finely chopped fresh mint**
- **1⅓ cups seeded and finely chopped cucumbers**
- **1⅓ cups seeded and finely chopped Roma tomatoes**
- **2 teaspoons finely chopped fresh parsley**
- **1 teaspoon fresh lemon juice**
- **1 teaspoon minced fresh garlic**
- **Pinch of salt**
- **¼ cup finely chopped red onion**
- **3 ounces reduced-fat feta cheese, crumbled**
- **2 tablespoons chopped Kalamata olives (about 8 olives)**
- **6 (about 6½-inch-diameter) whole-wheat pita circles, lightly toasted and cut into wedges**

Spoon the hummus into a 6-cup glass bowl. Use a spatula to spread it evenly to make one layer.

Mix the yogurt with the cumin and mint in a small bowl. Pour the yogurt mixture evenly over the hummus, and smooth it with the back of a spoon to form a second layer. Sprinkle the cucumbers evenly over the top.

Mix the tomatoes, parsley, lemon juice, garlic, and salt in a medium bowl. Sprinkle the tomato mixture over the cucumbers, followed by the onion, feta, then the olives.

Cover with plastic wrap and refrigerate for 1 to 6 hours. Serve with pita triangles for dipping.

> "Life is too short for a bad meal . . . but even shorter if you eat too many bad-for-you meals. So, I'm all about finding ways to indulge in the foods we all love without the excess fat and calories. There's nothing better than entertaining with healthier recipes and watching people enjoy food (and drinks!) that are actually good for them."
>
> **—Devin Alexander, author of The *Most Decadent Diet Ever!*, *Fast Food Fix*, and New York Times bestseller *The Biggest Loser Cookbook* and host of Healthy Decadence with Devin Alexander on Discovery Health and FitTV**

LYCHEE SNOW CONE

(Martini Glass)

If you have a taste for the exotic, this delectable concoction will bang your gong. Spoon it up as a snow cone or sip it with a straw as it melts. Either way, it is a unique addition to your Zen celebration.

Crushed ice

2 ounces lychee syrup

1 ounce passion fruit juice

½ ounce DRY Soda Co. Lemongrass soda

1 lychee

Using a large ice-cream scoop, put a ball of crushed ice into a martini glass. Mix the lychee syrup, fruit juice, and lemongrass soda, and drizzle it over the crushed ice. Top the snow cone ball with a lychee on a cocktail pick.

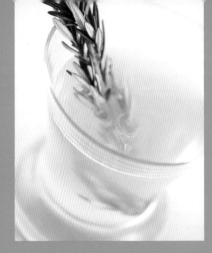

 PREGGIE PROVENÇE
(Cocktail Glass)

Reminiscent of the tranquil hillsides of southern France, this Preggatini pulls from fresh herb plants, lemon trees, grapevines, and lavender fields.

- **5–6 rosemary leaves**
- **3–4 white grapes, halved**
- **½ ounce simple syrup**
- **¼ teaspoon fresh lavender flower petals**
- **½ teaspoon grated lemon peel**
- **2 ounces lemonade**
- **3 ounces DRY Soda Co. Lavender soda**
- **1 lemon wheel**
- **1 sprig rosemary**

Muddle rosemary leaves with the cut grapes, simple syrup (recipe page 11), lavender flower petals, and grated lemon peel in the bottom of a mixing glass. Add lemonade, then shake well with ice. Strain into a cocktail glass. Top with lavender soda, and garnish with a lemon wheel and a sprig of rosemary.

De-Virginize for Dad ✎:
Use only 1 ounce lemonade, and add 1½ ounces rosemary-infused vodka.

Preggatini Punches

A great party requires good preparation. Assembling food and drink ahead of time makes entertaining a snap. These Preggatini Punches enable guests to serve themselves and are so pretty that they'll enhance your party buffet!

CITRUSY RED SANGRIA PUNCH
(Wine Goblet)

If you didn't discover Spanish sangria before the tapas craze, it is time to explore this popular Iberian export. Sangrias can be made any time of the year, with red or white wine, and feature whichever fruits are in season. Mamas-to-be can enjoy them, too, when nonalcoholic wine is substituted!

1 orange, cut into slices with peel on

1 lemon, cut into slices with peel on

1 lime, cut into slices with peel on

½ cup tangerine juice

½ cup pear cider

2 tablespoons sugar

2 bottles Fre Merlot alcohol-removed wine

Place cut fruit in a punch bowl, and stir in tangerine juice, pear cider, and sugar. Slowly add alcohol-removed wine. Cover and refrigerate at least 3 hours. Ladle it into wine goblets or punch cups when ready to serve.

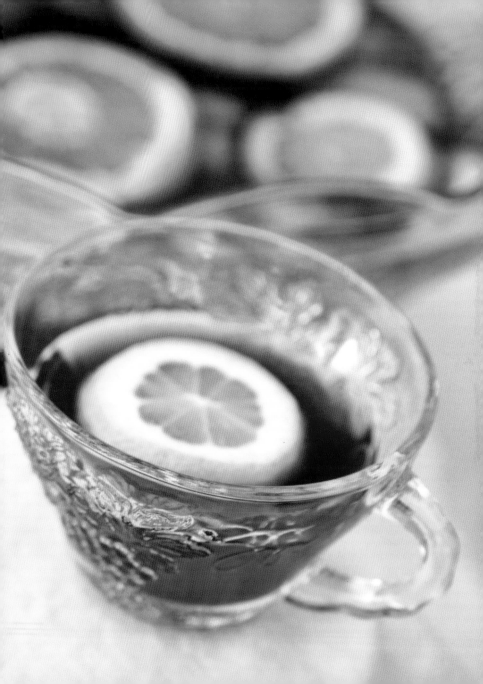

GINGER BELLINI PUNCH
(Wine Glass)

*The classic Bellini cocktail—created in Venice, Italy, in 1948—
recently celebrated its 60th anniversary. In this sparkling punch
version, I use a little ginger-infused simple syrup because it plays
nicely off the flavor of peach. (You may also have seen a rendition
of this recipe in the April 2008 issue of* Pregnancy *magazine.)*

- **1½ cups white peach puree (or peach nectar)**
- **⅓ cup ginger-infused simple syrup**
- **Juice from 1 lemon**
- **1 bottle nonalcoholic sparkling wine (or ¾ liter club soda)**
- **½ cup fresh raspberries**

Pour peach puree, ginger-infused simple syrup (recipe page
11), and lemon juice into a punch bowl. Stir. Slowly add alcohol-
removed sparkling wine (or club soda). Drop raspberries into the
punch for a burst of color. Serve in wine glasses.

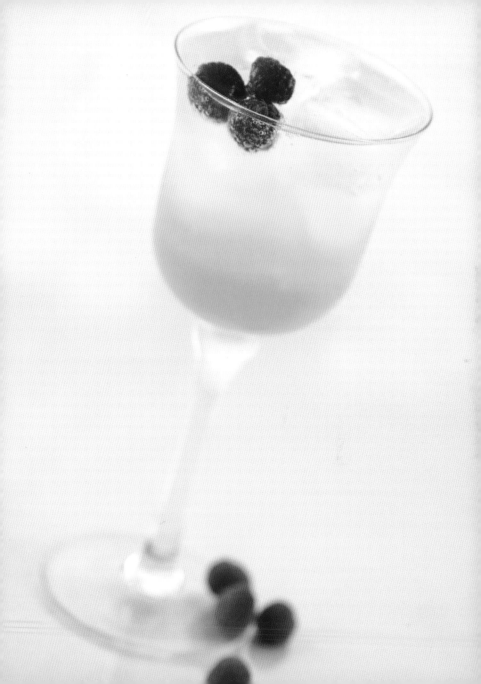

MINTY MANGO COOLER

(Tall Glass)

This punch tastes as good as it looks! Using fresh mint enhances both the flavor and the aroma.

2 cups white grape juice

3 cups mango nectar

1 bottle bitter lemon soda

3 trays mango-mint ice cubes*

2 bunches fresh mint

Pour white grape juice, mango nectar, and bitter lemon soda into a large pitcher or punch bowl. Add 1 tray of mango-mint ice cubes. To serve, place 2–3 fresh mango-mint ice cubes into a tall glass. Fill the glass with punch. Garnish each glass with a sprig of mint.

De-Virginize for Dad : Add 1 ounce Bacardi Peach Red rum or 1 ounce vodka.

Mango-Mint Ice Cubes

1½ cups mango juice

¼ cup water

¼ cup simple syrup (recipe page 11)

Juice from 1 lime

1 bunch mint leaves

Mix the first four ingredients, and pour into an ice cube tray. Place 1 mint leaf in each square. Freeze.

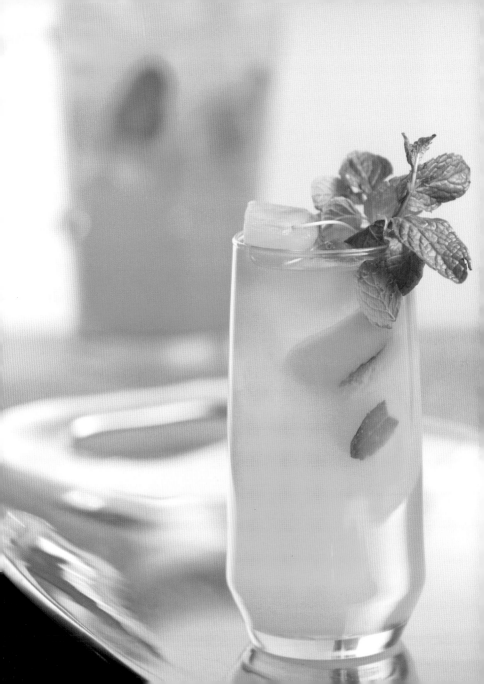

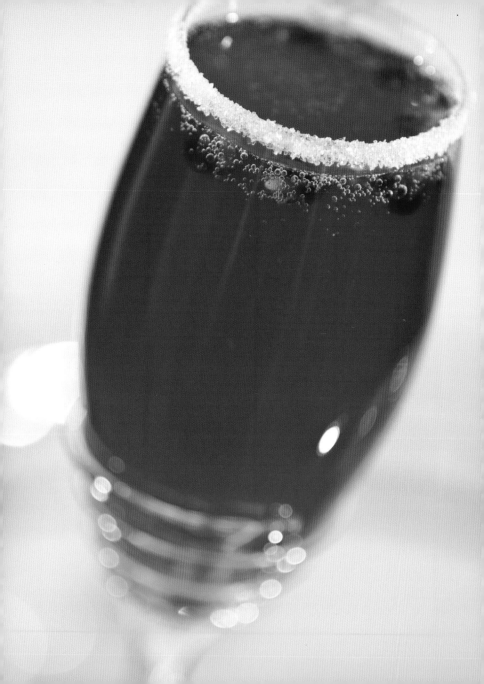

6

HOLIDAYS: CELEBRATE

No matter what time of year you're pregnant, you will encounter some holidays. Don't worry! Being booze-free doesn't mean being fun-free.

For those who normally (in a nonpregnant condition) would, oh, swig down a martini (or four) to deal with the pressure of hosting family gatherings 'round the turkey or planning a neighborhood Fourth of July picnic, don't sweat it! You will have a new form of "liquid courage" . . . your very own Holiday Preggatinis. Best of all, you can enlist well-intentioned but oh-so-meddlesome Aunt Myrtle to make them for you. (Once she's having a ball shaking, muddling, and mixing, she'll have less opportunity to give you all those unsolicited mothering tips, and you'll wind up with a refreshing beverage. It's a win-win situation.)

One of the many great things about being pregnant around any holiday is not feeling guilty indulging in extra helpings of all those special dishes people whip up only at certain times of the year. Nurturing family and friends will ply you with seconds of granny's coveted lasagna, your mom's nostalgic cheesecake, or your best friend's Christmas cookies—and won't it be liberating to say "Yes, please!" without worrying about your waistline?

Even better, while everyone else is guzzling spiked eggnog, sipping holiday-themed martinis, or making slurry champagne toasts on New Year's Eve, you can find solace in knowing that you will wake up without a hangover—or a fuzzy memory of Xeroxing your butt in the company copy room during the holiday party. Most of all, whichever holidays you mark while carrying that special delivery, you will have more to celebrate than ever before—your baby-to-be!

NEW YEAR'S DAY: BABY NEW YEAR BRUNCH PUNCH
(Wine Glass)

While everyone else has sagging eyes and a pounding head, you'll be as fresh as a daisy on January 1. You'll even have enough of this delicious alcohol-free champagne punch to share with those who overindulged the night before, proving that you truly are the bigger person. (Once into the third trimester, you just may be the bigger person regardless.)

2 cups freshly squeezed grapefruit juice
¼ cup simple syrup
Dash grapefruit bitters (optional)
2 bottles nonalcoholic sparkling wine
2 trays ruby red grapefruit–blueberry ice cubes*
Bouquet fresh lavender

Pour juice, simple syrup (recipe page 11), grapefruit bitters, and alcohol-removed sparkling wine into a punch bowl or large pitcher. Add 1 tray of grapefruit-blueberry ice cubes. To serve, place 1 fresh grapefruit-blueberry ice cube in each wine glass and fill with punch. Place the bouquet of fresh lavender near the punch bowl. Its calming smell helps soothe physical ailments, which may be comforting to hungover friends on New Year's Day!

*Ruby Red Grapefruit–Blueberry Ice Cubes (one tray)

2 cups grapefruit juice
Approx. 14 fresh blueberries

Fill an ice cube tray with the grapefruit juice, and place 1 blueberry in each square. Freeze.

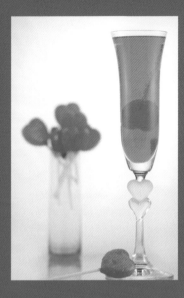

VALENTINE'S DAY: LOVE TRIANGLE
(Champagne Flute)

You may have never considered celebrating Valentine's Day as a threesome, until now. As baby snuggles in your belly, picture next year's romantic soiree: you clutching a screaming, squirming bundle of joy in one arm as you hold your husband's hand across a candlelit table with the other. "You + me + baby makes three" gives a whole new interpretation to the term love triangle!

1½ ounces white cranberry juice

¾ ounce Torani Strawberry syrup

2–3 drops grapefruit bitters (optional)

3 ounces nonalcoholic sparkling wine (or club soda)

Heart-shaped lollipops

Pour white cranberry juice, strawberry syrup, and bitters into a champagne flute. Top with alcohol-removed sparkling wine (or club soda). Garnish with a heart-shaped lollipop.

EASTER: SPARKLING CITRUS
(Champagne Flute)

Do you love your mimosas at Easter brunch? This Preggatini is a more exciting version of that post-Mass-and-Easter-egg-hunt, pre-all-you-can-eat-buffet interlude. Whether you are pregnant or simply abstaining from alcohol, this elegant sparkler tastes delicious and complements everything from Eggs Benedict to breakfast quiche.

Stirrings Tangerini Rimmer

2 ounces freshly squeezed pink grapefruit juice

1 ounce tangerine juice

Dash grapefruit bitters (optional)

2 ounces blood orange soda

Rim a champagne flute with rimming sugar. Pour in juices and dash of bitters, then top with blood orange soda.

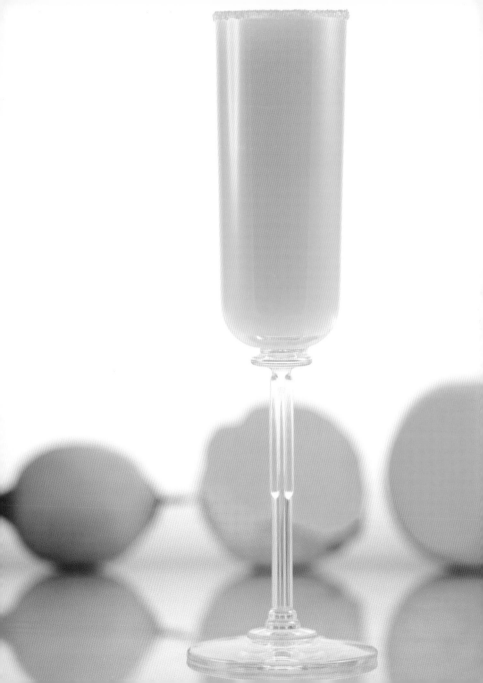

MOTHER'S DAY: THE PERFECT PEAR
(Martini Glass)

Whether celebrating your second month of pregnancy or your recent arrival, toast your partner with this perfect pear Preggatini to acknowledge the perfect pair you make.

Stirrings Pear Martini Rimmer

3 ounces pear nectar

½ ounce simple syrup

½ ounce lemon juice

2 ounces sparkling pear soda

1 edible flower

Rim a martini glass with pear rimmer and set aside. Pour pear nectar, simple syrup (recipe page 11), and lemon juice into a mixing glass, then add ice and shake. Strain into the rimmed martini glass. Top with sparkling pear soda. Gently lay an edible flower on the surface of the drink.

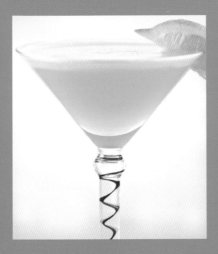

Y FATHER'S DAY: MY HONEYDEW
(Martini Glass)

"Honey do this, Honey do that . . ." will probably become common requests once the little one arrives and Mama needs an extra pair of hands. What better way to reward that strapping man for his hard work all year than by making him a refreshing cocktail you'll both enjoy?

- **½ cup honeydew melon chunks, seeded**
- **5–6 seedless white grapes, halved**
- **1 teaspoon fine sugar**
- **1 ounce lime juice**
- **Club soda**
- **1 lemon wedge**

Juice the melon chunks in a fruit juicer and set aside. Muddle grapes, sugar, and lime juice in the bottom of a mixing glass. Add ice and honeydew juice and shake vigorously. Strain into a martini glass, then top with club soda. Garnish with a lemon wedge.

De-Virginize for Dad 🍸: Add 1 ounce vodka and ½ ounce Midori melon liqueur.

FOURTH OF JULY: WATERMELON COOLER
(Wine Goblet)

What better to drink at a hot Independence Day picnic than the refreshing juice from America's favorite summertime melon? This colorful Preggatini will be the envy of all your nonpregnant friends!

6 mint leaves

1 heaping teaspoon powdered sugar

½ ounce lemon juice

Lemonade ice cubes (see page 102)

**1 cup seeded watermelon chunks
(to make approx. 4 ounces juice)**

2 ounces lemon-lime soda

1 watermelon wedge

Muddle mint, sugar, and lemon juice in the bottom of a wine goblet. Fill with lemonade ice cubes, add watermelon juice, and top with lemon-lime soda. Garnish with a watermelon wedge on the rim of the glass.

> *Take advantage of spring and summer fruits to create your own Preggatinis. Wild strawberries, peaches, melons, cherries, blackberries, and figs all make wonderful ingredients in both nonalcoholic and alcoholic cocktails.*

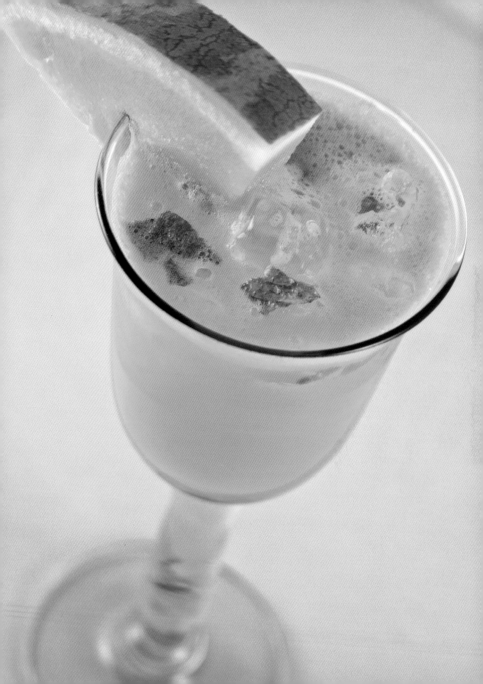

HALLOWEEN: GHOULISH GOBLET
(Wine Goblet)

This festive drink is a great nonalcoholic option for celebrating the spookiest night of the year. Your costume is already half-made if you decide to go as a naughty nun, Juno (from the 2007 blockbuster of the same name), or Katherine Heigl's character in Knocked Up!

1 skinny licorice rope

3 ounces blood orange juice

1½ ounces mango nectar

2 ounces blood orange soda

1 ounce grenadine

Coil a skinny licorice rope inside a wine goblet. Add blood orange juice, mango nectar, and ice. Top with blood orange soda. Gently pour in grenadine, letting it settle on the bottom of the glass.

De-Virginize for Dad : Gently pour in 1 ounce Blavod black vodka after the grenadine, to get a layered effect.

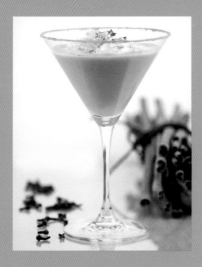

▼ THANKSGIVING: PUMPKIN PIE PREGGATINI
(Martini Glass)

If you love pumpkin pie, this Preggatini will remain a favorite long after the baby has arrived. Thick, creamy, and lip-smackingly decadent, it's practically a dessert unto itself. (This is one of my personal favorites year-round!)

- **2 graham crackers**
- **1 ounce Fee Brothers Spiced Cordial syrup**
- **2 ounces milk**
- **1½ ounces sweetened condensed milk**
- **1 heaping tablespoon canned pumpkin**
- **Dollop of whipped cream**

Grind graham crackers into fine crumbs in a food processor. Pour onto a small plate. On a separate plate, pour a small amount of spiced cordial syrup. Dip the rim of the martini glass into the syrup, then into the graham cracker crumbs, and set aside. Vigorously shake milk, sweetened condensed milk, remaining spiced cordial syrup, and pumpkin in a mixing glass with ice. Slowly strain into a rimmed martini glass. Top with a dollop of whipped cream.

HANUKKAH: BUBBLY BUBBALA

(Champagne Flute)

Menorah candles aren't the only things that sparkle during the Festival of Lights! This bubbly Preggatini snazzes up a special holiday celebration with your dear ones.

½ ounce simple syrup

½ ounce lemon juice

Sparkling concord grape juice

1 lemon wheel

Pour simple syrup (recipe page 11) and lemon juice into a champagne flute. Fill with sparkling concord grape juice. Garnish with a lemon wheel.

CHRISTMAS: SPICE OF THE SEASON MULLED WINE
(Bar Mug)

Simmering spiced wine on the stove makes the whole house smell like Christmas. With this alcohol-removed version, you don't have to miss out on that special aromatic memory (which may be amplified due to your heightened senses!)

1 bottle Fre Merlot alcohol-removed wine

1 teaspoon almond extract

2 cinnamon sticks*

3 whole cloves

½ teaspoon ground nutmeg

1 tablespoon honey

Pour wine into a double boiler over medium heat. Add all other ingredients, and stir until honey has dissolved. Reduce heat, cover, and gently simmer for 15 minutes, stirring occasionally. Serve in a bar mug.

*If desired, buy additional cinnamon sticks and garnish each cup with one.

NEW YEAR'S EVE: SPARKLING POMEGRANATE SNOWFLAKE
(Champagne Flute)

Top off a wonderful year with a special "champagne" cocktail. And just think: By this time next year, your baby will be celebrating with you!

2 tablespoons granulated, white sugar

1 sugar cube

Dash blood orange bitters

1½ ounces pomegranate juice

3 ounces nonalcoholic sparkling wine

1 teaspoon pomegranate seeds

Rim a champagne flute with sugar. Place the sugar cube into the bottom of the flute, and soak it with the bitters. Add pomegranate juice and alcohol-removed sparkling wine. Drop in pomegranate seeds.

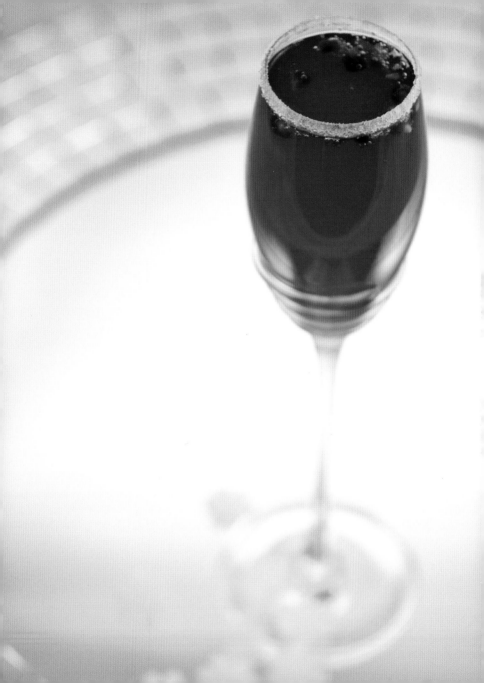

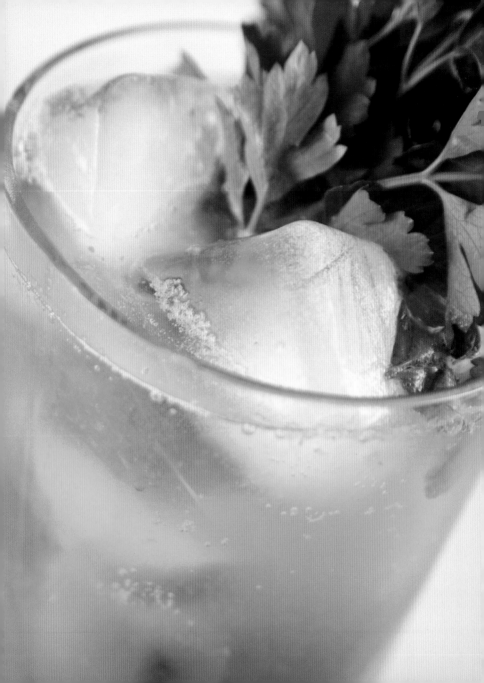

7

BREAST-FEEDING AND BEYOND: REINSTATE

Finally—the big moment is here. Yes, yes, the baby is wonderful, but I'm referring to getting the green light from your doctor to introduce small amounts of beer and wine back into everyday life. (Those who opt to forgo breast-feeding and use formula instead are completely in the clear!)

Of course you should follow your intuition on this issue. I don't advocate boozing it up while breast-feeding by any stretch of the imagination. The beer, wine, and sparkling wine options offered here can also be made with "near beer" and nonalcoholic wine and champagne if you prefer to continue to abstain completely.

However, with medical approval and a desire to dip a toe into the pond of luscious libations, the recipes in this chapter ease you back into imbibing. Additionally, for those already thinking about restoring their figures to pre-baby perfection, the low-calorie nonalcoholic Preggatinis in the last section of this chapter will help that effort!

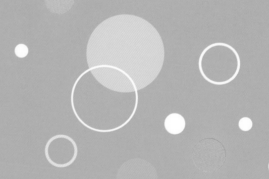

Beer Cocktails

The words beer and cocktail may seem contradictory, but they're not! Wonderful for summer barbeques or lounging by the lake, these cocktails dress up the average hot-dog-and-burger occasion. And, yes, men like them, too!

PANACHÉ
(Bar Mug)

Kissed with citrus and served ice-cold, this sunny refreshment is a favorite from the Mediterranean region.

4 ounces chilled beer

4 ounces bitter lemon soda

1 lemon wheel

Pour chilled beer and bitter lemon soda into an ice-filled beer mug. Garnish with a lemon wheel.

The Liquid Muse Mixology Tip: *To avoid too much foam when pouring beer from a bottle or tap, tilt the glass slightly so that the beer runs down the side of it rather than hitting the bottom of the glass directly.*

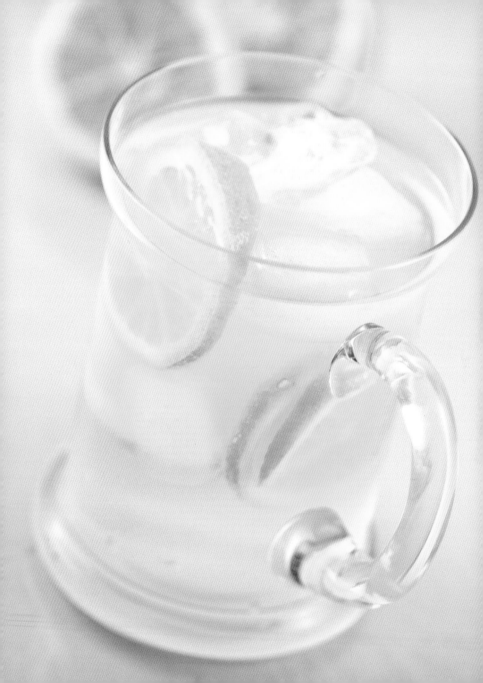

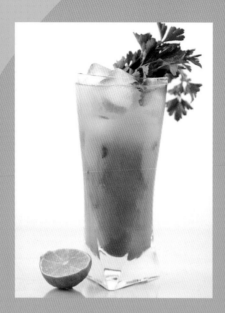

MEXICAN MICHELADA
(Bar Mug)

This brewed libation adds a splash of South of the Border flare to a backyard barbeque (great opportunity to show off the baby, of course) and brings a change of pace to taco night at home with the hubby.

4 ounces Clamato juice

½ ounce lemon juice

½ ounce lime juice

Dash Tabasco

Dash Worcestershire or soy sauce

4 ounces pale Mexican beer

1 leafy sprig cilantro

Pour juices and condiments into a chilled bar mug or tall glass. Add beer and stir. Garnish with cilantro.

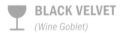

BLACK VELVET
(Wine Goblet)

Thick, creamy stout beer creates the bottom layer of this concoction, first dreamed up more than a century ago. Guinness is most commonly used, but you can experiment with any dark beer. Also try substituting hard cider for champagne.

4 ounces Guinness

4 ounces champagne

Slowly pour beer, then champagne, into a wine goblet.

> *Fact or Folklore? Although it is widely believed that a small amount of beer is a natural remedy to help a nursing mom's milk flow, others suggest that babies drink no alcohol-laced breast milk. It is advisable to get your doctor's opinion before you conduct your own experiment.*

Wine Cocktails

If you're a wine drinker, one of the biggest challenges during the last 40 weeks may have been giving up that playful pinot noir, forgoing your favorite spicy California zin, or turning down a glass of fancy French champagne. Now that you're ready to foray back into the vineyards, why not try a wine cocktail? Even winemakers who formerly cringed at the thought of anyone tinkering with vintages are reaching out to skilled mixologists.

FIRST CRUSH BLUSH
(Wine Glass)

Fruity and feminine, this wine spritzer gussies up a get-together with the girls.

3 strawberries, diced

1 ounce rose-infused simple syrup

3 ounces white zinfandel

Club soda

1 white rose

Muddle strawberries and rose-infused simple syrup (recipe page 11) in a mixing glass. Add ice and white zinfandel, and shake vigorously. Strain into a wine glass, and top with club soda. Garnish with a rose stem laid across the top of the glass.

"GREEN" AND WHITE SANGRIA
(Wine Glass)

This recipe is from The Liquid Muse "Sustainable Sips" organic cocktail class. It calls for one of my favorite California wines— Bonterra, made from organic grapes grown with sustainable farming methods. I suggest using Sauvignon Blanc because it has delightful hints of passion fruit and kiwi but the Chardonnay works well, too. I also marinate the chopped fruit in organic vodka because traditional red wine sangria often has a secondary liquor, such as brandy. However, that step is completely optional if you prefer to completely avoid hard liquor.

> **2 cups chopped seasonal organic fruits (e.g., strawberries and peaches in summer, figs and pears in winter)**
>
> **½ cup organic vodka (optional)**
>
> **¼ cup organic peach nectar**
>
> **2 bottles Bonterra Sauvignon Blanc**

Marinate chopped fruit in vodka and peach nectar for at least one hour in the refrigerator. When ready to serve, spoon a tablespoon of fruit mixture into a wine glass. Fill with ice, then top with wine. To prepare as a punch, place the fruit in a punch bowl, pour in peach nectar and wine. Chill for an hour, then let guests serve themselves.

THE LIQUID MUSE CHAMPAGNE COCKTAIL
(Champagne Flute)

I love champagne with just about anything! When I combined it with port to make my version of a traditional champagne cocktail, I knew I'd found something I'd serve again and again.

1 sugar cube

Dash Fee Brothers Whiskey Barrel bitters

1 ounce port

4 ounces champagne

1 orange peel twist

Douse a sugar cube with bitters, and drop it into the bottom of a champagne flute. Add port and champagne. Garnish with an aromatic orange peel twist.

> *Fact or Fiction? Grapes must be grown organically and/or sustainably for a minimum of three years before a winery can declare itself organic. While organic farming keeps chemicals from touching the grapes, do not believe the hype that drinking organic equals no hangover. The only way to avoid dehydration and a pounding head is to drink plenty of water and imbibe alcohol in moderation!*

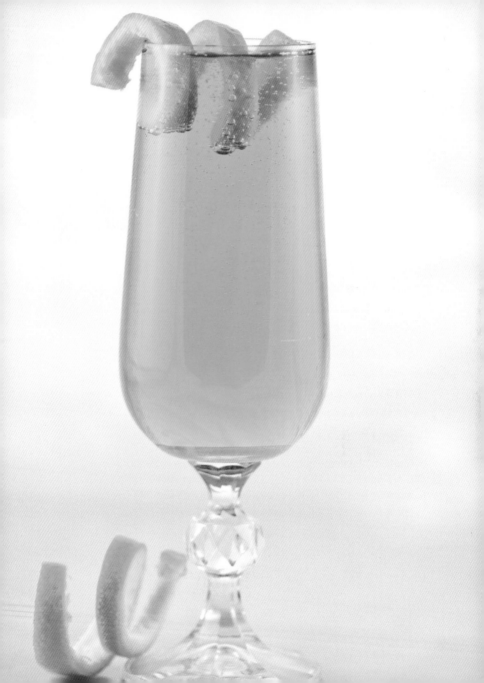

Low-Calorie Preggatinis

Most women gain 25–40 pounds during pregnancy. Once the little one pops out, however, a new mom wants to get back to her original form as soon as possible! Although breast-feeding is nature's way of burning extra calories, a little exercise and diet awareness definitely help the cause. I've limited the calories in these Preggatinis so you can work them into your daily regimen.

HOT MAMA Approx. 52 calories
(Martini Glass)

Hot peppers not only spice up your love life as natural aphrodisiacs, they also rev up your metabolism!

4 slices jalapeño

½ ounce lime juice

3 drops grapefruit bitters

3 ounces orange juice

2 ounces diet ginger ale

Muddle 1 jalapeño slice, lime juice, and bitters in the bottom of a mixing glass. Add orange juice and ice, then shake. Strain into a martini glass. Top with diet ginger ale. Garnish with the remaining jalapeño slices floating on the surface of the drink.

SKINNY MINNIE PREGGATINI Approx. 41 calories
(Tall Glass)

Grapefruits are so hailed for their fat-burning benefits that there is a whole diet fad created around them. This drink is by no means a meal replacement but rather an enhancement to any diet plan.

2 sections grapefruit, peeled

Dash grapefruit bitters

½ ounce lemon juice

1½ ounces grapefruit juice

3 ounces diet tonic water

Muddle grapefruit, bitters, and lemon juice in the bottom of a tall glass. Add ice and grapefruit juice. Top with diet tonic water.

🍸 **The Liquid Muse Mixology Tip:** *An ounce of alcohol has roughly 70–90 calories. Add that into the total calorie count for "De-Virginize for Dad" options, in case your man was a good sport during your pregnancy and packed on a few extra pounds in solidarity.*

COSMOMPOLITAN COOLER Approx. 43 calories
(Tall Glass)

With a flavor profile similar to everyone's favorite Cosmopolitan, this cooler has fewer calories than a chocolate chip cookie!

2 ounces cranberry juice

1 ounce lime juice

½ ounce Stirrings Blood Orange bitters

4 ounces lime-flavored sparkling water

1 lime wedge

Fill a tall glass with ice, and pour in all liquid ingredients. Stir with a bar spoon. Garnish with a wedge of lime.

If the average baby weighs 7½ pounds, why does the average pregnant lady gain at least 30 pounds? Women carry about 4 extra pounds of additional blood and about 25 pounds of other fluids and tissue while the baby is growing.

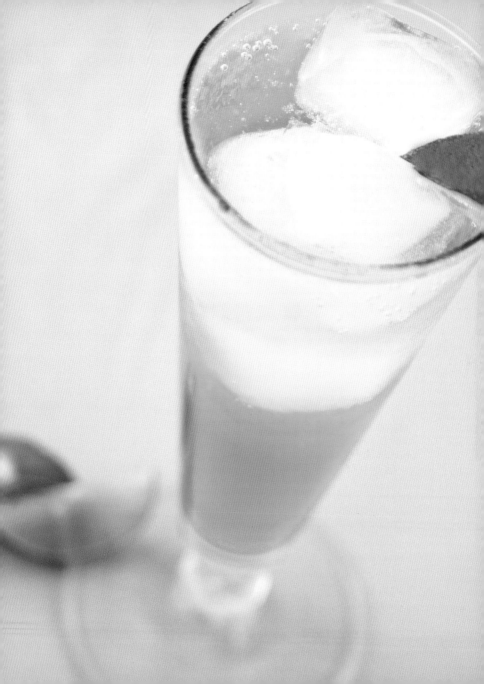

Index

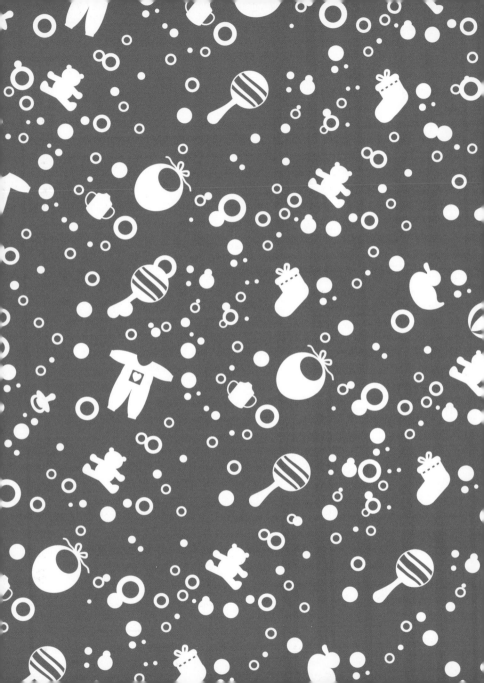